SPEECH DISORDERS

RESOURCE GUIDE FOR PRESCHOOL CHILDREN

SINGULAR RESOURCE GUIDE SERIES

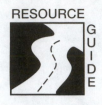

EDITOR

Ken Bleile, Ph.D.
Department of Communicative Disorders
University of Northern Iowa
Cedar Falls, Iowa

ASSOCIATE EDITORS

Brian Goldsein, Ph.D.
Communications Sciences
Temple University
Philadelphia, Pennsylvania

Sharron Glennen, Ph.D.
Department of Communication Sciences and Disorders
Towson University
Towson, Maryland

Carole Roth, Ph.D.
Department of Speech Pathology
Hennepin County Medical Center
Minneapolis, Minnesota

Amy Weiss, Ph.D.
Department of Speech Pathology and Audiology
University of Iowa
Iowa City, Iowa

Tricia Zebrowski, Ph.D.
Department of Speech Pathology and Audiology
University of Iowa
Iowa City, Iowa

SPEECH DISORDERS

RESOURCE GUIDE FOR PRESCHOOL CHILDREN

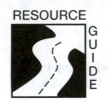

A. Lynn Williams, Ph.D.
East Tennessee State University

THOMSON
DELMAR LEARNING

Australia   Canada   Mexico   Singapore   Spain   United Kingdom   United States

THOMSON
* * *
DELMAR LEARNING

i 0 769 300 804

NOTICE TO THE READER

Publisher does not warrant or guarantee any of the products described herein or perform any independent analysis in connection with any of the product information contained herein. Publisher does not assume, and expressly disclaims, any obligation to obtain and include information other than that provided to it by the manufacturer.

The reader is expressly warned to consider and adopt all safety procedures that might be indicated by the activities herein and to avoid all potential hazards. By following the instructions contained herein, the reader willingly assumes all risks in connection with such hazards.

The Publisher makes no representation or warranties of any kind, including but not limited to the warranties of fitness for particular purpose or merchantability, nor are such representations implied with respect to the material set forth herein, and the publisher takes no responsibility with respect to such material. The publisher shall not be liable for any special, consequential, or exemplary damages resulting, in whole or part, from the readers' use of, or reliance upon, this material.

Executive Director, Health Care Business Unit:
William Brottmiller

Executive Editor:
Cathy L. Esperti

Acquisitions Editor:
Candice Janco

Developmental Editor:
Patricia A. Gaworecki

COPYRIGHT © 2003 Delmar Learning. Singular Publishing Group is an imprint of Delmar Learning, a division of Thomson Learning, Inc. Thomson Learning ™ is a trademark used herein under license.

Printed in United States of America

1 2 3 4 5 6 7 XXX 06 05 04 03 02

For more information, contact Singular Publishing Group Executive Woods 5 Maxwell Drive Clifton Park, NY 12065-2919; or find us on the World Wide Web at:
http://www.delmarhealthcare.com

Editorial Assistant:
Maria D'Angelico

Executive Marketing Manager:
Dawn F. Gerrain

Channel Manager:
Jennifer McAvey

ALL RIGHTS RESERVED. No part of this work covered by the copyright hereon may be reproduced or used in any form or by any means— graphic, electronic, or mechanical, including photocopying, recording, taping, Web distribution, or information storage and retrieval systems—without the written permission of the publisher.

For permission to use material from this text or product, contact us by
Tel (800) 730-2214
Fax (800) 730-2215
www.thomsonrights.com

Production Editor:
James Zayicek

ISBN 0-7693-0080-4

Library of Congress Cataloging-in-Publication Data
Williams, A. Lynn
Speech disorders resource guide for
preschool children / A. Lynn Williams
p. cm.—(Singular resource guide series)
Includes index.
ISBN 0-7693-0080-4
1. Speech disorders in children. 2. Language disorders in children.
I. Title. II. Series.

RJ496.S7 W47 2003
61892'855—dc21
2002067577

CONTENTS

SECTION 1: CORE KNOWLEDGE   1

SECTION 2: ASSESSMENT PROCEDURES   25

SECTION 3: ANALYSIS PROCEDURES — 47

SECTION 4: INTERVENTION PRINCIPLES, METHODS, AND MODELS — 81

SECTION 5: PHONOLOGICAL AWARENESS AND SPEECH DISORDERS — 127

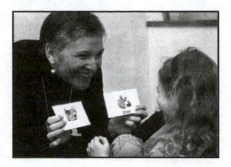

ABOUT THE AUTHOR

A. Lynn Williams, Ph.D., CCC-SLP, is a professor in the Department of Communicative Disorders at East Tennessee State University in Johnson City, Tennessee. Her extensive clinical background serves as a foundation for her work with children who have speech disorders. Her research and practice have focused on developing assessment and intervention models that utilize linguistic methodology and principles to describe disordered sound systems and to facilitate sound learning through the manipulation of the systematic and functional properties of the child's sound system. Dr. Williams has developed a model for phonological intervention called multiple oppositions that is the basis for several presentations and publications. She recently completed a phonological intervention study on multiple oppositions that was funded by the National Institutes of Health. Dr. Williams is currently developing a software program for phonological intervention called *Sound Contrasts in Phonology (SCIP)*, which is designed to help clinicians access resources for utilization in the newer models of phonological intervention.

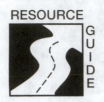

FOREWORD

The emblem for this series is a stylized road map. This symbol is intended to represent the goal of the series: to create books that serve as road maps to the care of communicative disorders. Like good road maps, each book gives the clinician an honest depiction of the territory, shows the various routes, and enables you, the traveler, to select the route best suited for your particular type of journey. Each book's author is someone who knows the territory about which he or she is writing, both as a clinician and as a researcher. The hope of all involved in this series is that you will find the books useful and readable. Good traveling!

Ken Bleile, Ph.D.

PREFACE

Things do not change; we change.
Henry David Thoreau

The area of clinical phonology is in a dynamic period of growth and expansion. In the last decade, tremendous advances and development of theoretical orientations, assessment procedures, and intervention models have been published and debated. As clinicians, we are faced with new ideas to consider and information to integrate into clinical application. The idea of creating a resource guide to address the enormous changes in this area was very appealing to me. This resource guide was written for students and practicing clinicians who want to keep current with the intellectual pace of these recent advances, especially for individuals who are expected to deal with many different types of disorders and have limited time for reading the literature or attending workshops.

My goal in writing this book was to provide a comprehensive resource guide for working with young children who have disordered sound systems. While this text is armed specifically at working with the preschool-aged child, the many tools and resources found in this book can be used with children up to eight years old. Specifically, my objectives in this book included:

1. To provide a foundation for understanding disordered speech and reviewing the tools of phonetic transcription and classification that are prerequisite to our clinical assessments and interventions of speech disorders

2. To provide resources for available tests, procedures, and components of a phonological/speech assessment

3. To describe a variety of phonological analyses in a step-by-step fashion that can be used to analyze disordered speech

4. To describe a broad range of articulatory and phonological intervention approaches in sufficient detail that will enable clinicians to choose and implement the most appropriate treatment approach

5. To present information about the assessment and treatment of phonological awareness skills

6. To present procedures for assessing treatment efficacy that will assist clinicians with demonstrating accountability and evaluating treatment outcomes

We have the remarkable challenge and opportunity to make a difference in children's lives who have disordered sound systems. I hope the information presented in this book provides a useful resource to the readers in their work with these children.

ACKNOWLEDGMENTS

It is good to have an end to journey towards; but it is the journey that matters in the end.
Ursula K. LeGuin

I have had the very competent support of several capable people along the journey of writing this book. A primary influence in the formation of this book was Ken Bleile. He had the insight and vision for the Resource Guide series and had faith in my abilities to write this book for young children who have speech disorders. I am thankful to him for leading me on this wonderful journey. I value the guidance provided by the thoughtful and insightful reviews completed by Amy Weiss, Brian Goldstein, and Ken Bleile. Their comments regarding both style and content added to the clarity and readability of the book. Finally, I appreciate the calm encouragement of Patty Gaworecki at Delmar Learning, especially regarding deadlines.

I am fortunate to have had the opportunity to work with creative and bright students over the years who have stretched my thinking about the assessment and treatment of speech disorders in children. Their questions and discussions clarified many of my ideas and hypotheses. Several of these students were directly involved in helping me put this book together. Special thanks goes to Amanda Lambert Rowland, Krista Lowe, Traci Van Nostran, and Tracy Ford for their help in finding references and typing tables. I am particularly grateful to Lisa Cooper and Cami Huff for their help in the final phases of the book. They kept everything, including me, from coming unglued.

To the children and their families, I am especially indebted. I am continually amazed at the creative, logical, and unique abilities that children have in developing their sound systems. Every child has presented me with a distinctive opportunity and challenge to discover "the order in the disorder." I have learned a great deal from the wisdom of many parents who have shared their child's "own language" with me.

All of these individuals have helped me with the vision of this book. It was, however, my community of family who made the vision a reality. I appreciate the summers that my parents, Nita and Billo Williams, cared for my children while I wrote. My greatest appreciation and gratitude go to my husband, Jim Bitter, and our daughters, Alison and Nora. Their unending patience, encouragement, and support were essential for the professional journey that I undertook in writing this book.

DEDICATION

To Jim, Alison, and Nora

with love and affection

SECTION

CORE KNOWLEDGE

· ·

"Phonological disorders arise more in the mind than in the mouth." (Grunwell, 1987)

SETTING THE STAGE

There have been considerable changes over the years in the way children's speech disorders have been assessed and treated. The introduction of phonological principles from the field of linguistics was responsible for many of these changes. Although the terms and concept of phonology have existed in our literature for more than two decades, many speech-language pathologists (SLPs) continue to express confusion over the use of phonological terms and principles as well as uncertainty about the benefits of incorporating a phonological approach into their clinical practice. This confusion and uncertainty is mirrored in Hodson's (1992) estimate that only about 10% of practicing SLPs in the United States and Canada utilize phonological principles in their clinical practices with children who have speech disorders.

The changes and developments in the area of child speech disorders are also apparent in defining speech disorders. We will use the broader term "speech disorders" in this text to include both articulation and phonological disorders. Traditionally, articulation disorder referred to speech disorders that are phonetic and related to the peripheral aspects of sound production. Phonological disorder, however, has also been used to describe many of the same children who were previously described as having an articulation disorder. The difficulty with these terms is that a given child with a speech disorder might exhibit both articulatory and phonologic errors. Elbert (1992) and others have suggested that a speech disorder that has been diagnosed as phonologic can also have a phonetic, or articulatory, component.

1

Thus, we will use the broader term "speech disorders," which includes speech errors that can be phonetic, phonemic, or both. This term acknowledges the interrelated and interdependent nature of articulation and phonology. It concedes the dual nature of the phonology of a language in which the acquisition of a sound system includes an inventory of sounds that are used contrastively to signal meaning differences, a set of rules that specify the permissible combinations of sounds and distribution of sounds within a language, as well as the processes involved in the planning and execution of motor sequences of the peripheral speech mechanism to produce the speech sounds. With this term, speech disorders include speech disabilities that arise from either a peripheral or central level, or both, given that a problem in the central, cognitive-phonological processing level would impact the peripheral level of sound production as well (Williams, 2001).

Characteristics of a Speech Disorder

From a phonological perspective, Grunwell (1997) described the characteristics of a speech disorder in terms of system, structure, and stability. Specifically, the child's sound *system* is smaller than the adult system in which there is an absence of adult sound contrasts. This absence results in phoneme collapses (Williams, 2000), in which the child produces one sound for several different adult sounds. For example, the child produces [t] for /t, k, tʃ, s, and ʃ/, which results in homonymous pronunciations of [tɪp] for "tip," "Kip," "chip," "sip," and "ship." Williams (2000) described these phoneme collapses as compensatory strategies that the child has developed in order to accommodate his or her limited, or smaller, sound system relative to the larger adult sound system. As such, there is a relationship between the phonetic properties of the collapsed adult targets and the child's errored substitution. In the previous example, the child collapsed voiceless obstruents /t, k, tʃ, s, and ʃ/ to a voiceless obstruent [t] that was available in his or her sound system.

With regard to *structure*, Grunwell (1997) described the child's phonotactic patterns as being more simplistic relative to the structure of the adult sound system. For example, children who have speech disorders frequently simplify the more complex adult structure of consonant clusters to a singleton (for example, "stop" produced as [tɑp]).

In terms of *stability*, Grunwell (1997) stated that there is a tendency for some variability in the child's realizations of the adult target. For example, the child might sometimes produce target /k/ as [t] or [g]. This variability might be based on position in the word or syllable in which the target occurs, or it could be influenced by the vowel environment, as in complementary distribution.

Notice that none of the characteristics of a speech disorder involve any defects of the speech or hearing mechanisms or of the central and peripheral nervous systems. In this regard, speech disorders are referred to as *functional*, which means that there is no organic basis for the speech disorder.

In summary, many speech disorders in children are characterized by a limited sound system in which there is a relationship between the phonetic properties of the child's production and the intended target(s). It is more simplistic in structure, and there is a tendency for some variability in the child's system relative to the adult sound system that might be rule-based or free variation as the child revises his or her sound system.

Classification of Speech Disorders

In an attempt to understand the nature of speech disorders in children, researchers have proposed classifications or typologies of speech disorders (cf., Ingram, 1997; Shriberg, 1982 and

TABLE 1–1   Classification of Speech Disorders in Children (Shriberg, 1997)

Special Populations	Speech Delay	Residual Errors
speech-hearing mechanism; cognitive-linguistic processes; psychosocial processes	deletion/substitution errors	distortion errors of fricatives, affricates, and/or liquids
birth to beyond age 9	birth to age 9	older children ($\geq$ 9 years)
	concomitant language impairment	

1994). Most notable is the work of Shriberg and his colleagues to describe three populations of childhood speech disorders (Shriberg, 1997) (Table 1–1). Shriberg described these three populations as residual errors (RE), speech delay (SD), and special populations (SP). Children who form the population of residual errors are typically older children who have retained a few speech sound errors beyond the typical developmental period of acquisition. Their errors are typically distortions of fricatives, affricates, and/or liquids.

SD includes children from a larger developmental period that spans from birth to about nine years of age. Children in this population exhibit deletion and substitution errors beyond those observed in their typically developing-age peers. The severity of the speech disorder in this group is greater than in the RE population in that the errors of children in this group impact the intelligibility of their speech. In addition, these children also frequently exhibit concomitant language impairment that also impacts their academic abilities.

The third population of speech disorders in children is the category "SP." Unlike the children in the two previous groups of unknown origin of the speech disorder, these children have special needs in health or educational areas. Shriberg and Kwiatkowski (1994) classified the SP group into three subgroups based on etiology: speech-hearing mechanism, cognitive-linguistic processes, and psychosocial processes. The speech disorders of children in the SP category can span the age period from birth to beyond the typical nine-year age level for normal phonological acquisition.

Prevalence and Significance of Speech Disorders in Children

Speech disorders are a widespread problem in preschool and school-age children. Approximately 10–15% of preschoolers and about 6% of school-age children in grades 1–12 exhibit a speech disorder (American Speech-Language-Hearing Association, 2000; Bello, 1995). Further concern about the incidence of speech disorders in this age group includes recent research on the correlation between phonological disorders and academic difficulties. Specifically, 50% to 70% of the children with phonological disorders exhibit general academic difficulty throughout high school (Felsenfeld, Broen, and McGue, 1994; Shriberg and Kwiatkowski, 1988). The academic difficulties stem from the high correlation between phonological disorders and difficulties with written language, including reading, writing, spelling, and mathematics (Bird, Bishop, and Freeman, 1995; Catts, 1993; Clark-Klein and Hodson, 1995). Finally, many children with phonological disorders also experience socialization difficulties (cf., Rice, Hadley, and Alexander, 1993). Follow-up studies have reported that 54% of parents rated their children as exhibiting social competence problems and 70% as having behavioral problems 10 years after their children were initially diagnosed in preschool as language impaired (Aram and Hall, 1989).

Given the incidence and related problems associated with speech disorders, there is a significant need and interest in incorporating models of assessment and intervention that are effective and efficient in increasing speech intelligibility. The urgency in understanding speech disorders and applying efficacious intervention programs is further highlighted by the notion of a critical period hypothesis. Bishop and Adams (1990) asserted that written language skills (reading, writing, and spelling) will progress normally as long as the speech impairment has been resolved by 5 years, 6 months.

Legal Precedence

The provision of clinical services (assessment and intervention) to children with speech disorders are mandated by two pieces of federal legislation. The Education for All Handicapped Children Act (PL 94-142) enacted in 1975 mandates free and appropriate education to all children with handicaps from ages 3 to 21. This education includes a thorough assessment to determine the nature and degree of the disability, educational services that are implemented to the specific needs of the child, educational placement in the least restrictive environment, and provision of any supplementary resource services that are needed to ensure the child's success in school.

The second piece of federal legislation is PL 99-457 Part H, which extended the provision of services to children from birth to three years of age. According to Safer and Hamilton (1993), the enactment of PL 99-457 in 1986 (changed by PL 101-476 to the Individuals with Disabilities Education Act, or IDEA) was the culmination of a movement that began with the pioneering efforts of program developers and researchers who demonstrated the long-lasting benefits and lower costs of providing early intervention services for young children and their parents. IDEA has been described as watershed legislation that has as important and far-reaching benefits for young children and their families as PL 94-142 had for school-age children and their families. Children who are eligible for services under PL 99-457 are those who are experiencing developmental delays in one or more developmental domains (physical, cognitive, communicative, social or emotional, or adaptive development) or who have a diagnosed physical or mental condition that has a high probability of resulting in developmental delay. Under this legislation, families are viewed as playing a key role in the development of the young child. Families are regarded as the most knowledgeable individuals regarding their children, as a constant in a child's life, and as the provider of stimulation and emotional support. This family-oriented perspective is reflected in the *individualized family service plan* (IFSP) that specifies the delivery of services. Part of the legislation of 99-457 therefore focused on the needs of the family with a responsibility to support the family.

TERMINOLOGY

Some general terms are defined in this section that are important to the assessment and intervention of speech disorders in children. More specific terminology is defined in the glossary that is included at the end of the book.

> **Abbreviations**—letters will be used throughout this book to represent different phonetic or linguistic phenomena. These abbreviations will include the following:
>
> **C** (consonant)   **WI** (word-initial)
>
> **V** (vowel)   **WF** (word-final)
>
> **S** (syllable)

Grapheme—orthographic letters that comprise the alphabetic writing system. Letters are not to be confused with phonetic symbols.

IPA—International Phonetic Alphabet, which contains the symbols to represent the sounds in all natural languages of the world. Phonetic symbols are not to be confused with graphemes, or letters.

Linguistic notation—linguistic abbreviations will be used throughout this book to represent positions of sounds within words and syllables. These abbreviations will include the following:

# ___	word-initial
___ #	word-final
V___V	intervocalic
V ___	post-vocalic

Other linguistic notation will be used to write phonological rules. The basic notation for rules is $X \rightarrow Y / $___ , which states that "X goes to Y in the environment of." This relationship can be thought of as a shorthand to characterize children's phonological rules or error patterns. To illustrate the linguistic notation for the phonological rule of word-final consonant deletion, the rule would be written as follows:

$C \rightarrow \emptyset / $___ #

Phonological disorder—a specific term used to describe errored patterns of speech that reflect a linguistic, or phonemic, disorder in which the speech difficulties arise from differences in the development of phonological rules and in phonological organization relative to the ambient, or target, speech community

Speech delay—a term used to describe the slower speech development in children; generally about a year's delay

Speech differences—differences in speech that are characteristic of a particular linguistic or cultural group and are not considered a speech disorder

Speech disorder—a generic term used to describe both the phonetic and phonemic aspects of speech disorders in children

PHONETIC TRANSCRIPTION

Hodson (1992) claimed that only about 10% of SLPs incorporated phonological principles into their assessment and intervention practices with children who have functional speech disorders. She suggested one reason for this low practice rate is a lack of training in phonetic transcription and classification. Phonetic transcription is a tool skill of the profession. Similar to any skill, "If you don't use it, you lose it." Too often, students trained in communicative disorders complete their phonetics coursework two to three years before they begin their clinical practice. Depending on their caseloads and the preferences and clinical orientation of their clinical supervisors, they might be required to only use a limited aspect of their phonetics training. Based on the orientation toward speech disorders in children in previous decades, a simple plus-or-minus (+/−) scoring system on sound inventory tests was sufficient for assessing a child's productions. It has only been in recent years that whole-word transcriptions on these tests have been recommended or required in order to complete any type of phonological analysis of the child's single-word responses. This situation being the case, better skills with the use of phonetic transcription are needed.

A brief review of phonetic transcription is provided. Readers, however, are referred to Shriberg and Kent (1995) for a more complete reference of the classification and transcription of English consonants and vowels. Our analyses of a child's sound system can only be as informative as our transcriptions are accurate. If our transcriptions are incorrect, then so will be our analysis of the child's phonology. Taking this situation one step further, our intervention can only be as efficacious as our analyses are accurate. Thus, treatment efficacy begins with accurate phonetic transcriptions and classification of the child's sound inventory and rules relative to the adult sound system.

Consonant and Vowel Classification: A Review

Consonants and vowels can be described according to two different classifications: (1) traditional classification of place, voice, and manner for consonants or tongue height, tongue advancement, lip rounding, and tension for vowels; and (2) distinctive features. Most SLPs are trained to describe English phonemes according to the traditional classification. Recently, however, with the incorporation of more linguistic methods of describing and treating disordered sound systems, consonants and vowels are described according to the distinctive feature classification system. A quick review of both classification systems will be given for consonants and vowels.

Consonants: Traditional Classification

The traditional classification describes the production of consonants along three broad parameters of production: (1) place of production; (2) manner of production; and (3) voicing. Place of production describes *where* in the vocal tract the sound is produced. Manner of production describes *how* the sound is produced. Voicing describes whether or not the sound is produced with vocal fold vibration.

There are seven places of English consonant production. Moving from the most anterior to the most posterior places of production, these include:

1. bilabial—sounds produced with both lips [p, b, m, w*]

   * [w] involves two places of articulation and is thus more accurately described as a labio-velar place of production.

2. labio-dental—sounds produced with the upper teeth and lower lip [f, v]

3. lingua-dental—sounds produced with the tongue between the teeth [θ, ð].

   These symbols are frequently referred to as "theta" for the voiceless [θ] and "eth" for the voiced [ð].

4. alveolar—sounds produced with tongue-tip elevation at the alveolar ridge [t, d, s, z, n, l]

5. palatal—sounds produced in the region of the hard palate [ʃ, ʒ, tʃ, dʒ, j, r].

   The symbols [ʃ, ʒ] are referred to as "esh" and "ezh," respectively. The symbols [tʃ, dʒ] are referred to as "etch" and "edge," respectively.

6. velar—sounds produced in the region of the soft palate [k, g, ŋ].

   The symbol [ŋ] is referred to as "ang."

7. glottal—sounds produced at the level of the glottis [h, ʔ]

There are six manner categories of English consonant production. These include:

1. stops—sounds produced with a complete obstruction of the vocal tract
   [p, b, t, d, k, g, ʔ]

2. fricatives—sounds produced with a partial obstruction of the vocal tract
   [f, v, θ, ð, s, z, ʃ, ʒ] and [h] according to some classifications. Due to the limited distribution of [h] to word-initial and word-medial positions, it is often classified as a glide rather than a fricative.

3. affricates—sounds produced with a brief constriction of the vocal tract and then a gradual release of the airstream [tʃ, dʒ]

4. nasals—sounds produced with the velopharyngeal port open, which allows for nasal resonance [m, n, ŋ]

5. glides—sounds produced with a gliding movement of the tongue toward or from a vowel [w, j, h]. These sounds have a limited distribution in that they can only occur at the beginning or middle of words, never at the end. For this reason, [h] is often classified as a glide rather than a fricative.

6. liquids—sounds produced with a relatively open vocal tract that is only somewhat more restricted than that for vowels [l, r]. These sounds can function as either consonants or vowels.

English consonants can be classified as either voiced or voiceless. Voicing refers to the presence or absence of vocal fold vibration during the production of a sound. The following sounds are listed according to their voicing characteristics:

	Voiced	*Voiceless*
stops	[b, d, g]	[p, t, k, ʔ]
fricatives	[v, ð, z, ʒ]	[f, θ, s, ʃ, h]
affricates	[dʒ]	[tʃ]
nasals	[m, n, ŋ]	
glides	[w, j]	[h]
liquids	[l, r]	

It is easier to describe the voicing contrast in terms of pairs of sounds that are identical in place and manner characteristics but that differ only in voicing (Table 1–2). These sounds are called cognates. Notice that there are only voicing pairs, or cognates, in the stop, fricative, and affricate categories. The last three manner categories of nasals, glides, and liquids did not have any voiceless sounds with the exception of [h], which is dually classified as a fricative and only characterized as a glide on the basis of its distribution limitations.

This voicing difference between the top three manner categories (stops, fricatives, and affricates) and the last three manner classes of sounds (nasals, glides, and liquids) represents one of the major distinctions between these two groups of sounds. Stops, fricatives, and affricates comprise the group of sounds referred to as *obstruents*. These sounds are similar in that each is produced with complete or partial obstruction of the vocal tract, and they can be produced with or without vocal fold vibration. Conversely, nasals, glides, and liquids comprise the group of

TABLE 1–2

	Bilabial	Linguadental	Labiodental	Alveolar	Palatal	Velar	Glottal
Stops	p b			t d		k g	ʔ
Fricatives		θ ð	f v	s z	ʃ ʒ		h
Affricates					tʃ dʒ		
Nasals	m			n		ŋ	
Liquids				l	r		
Glides	w*				j	w*	h

* indicates labio-velar place of production

sounds referred to as *sonorants*. These sounds are produced with little or no vocal tract obstruction and all are produced with spontaneous voicing so that there are no voiceless sounds. This distinction of obstruent-sonorant represents a major class distinction in distinctive features, as we will discuss later. Traditional classification of the consonants is summarized in the following chart. Notice that the top three manner classes of sounds (stops, fricatives, and affricates) are separated from the last three manner classes of sounds (nasals, liquids, and glides) to indicate the obstruent-sonorant distinction. Also notice the dual classification of [h] as a fricative and a glide based on the distributional characteristics of [h], which we discussed previously.

The three parameters of place, voice, and manner can be used to describe a class of sounds, as described earlier, or can be combined to describe a single sound. For example, a voiceless bilabial stop describes the sound [p]. Voiceless stops describe a larger group of sounds ([p, t, k, ʔ]). It is important to learn the characteristics of place, voice, and manner of each of the English consonants; however, it is important to understand each of these parameters so you know the classification of consonants in a multidimensional rather than in a rote, unidimensional way. It is important to be able to recombine these parameters into different arrangements and find the commonality among a group of sounds. For example, what is common about the group of sounds [d, z, n, l]? If your answer is that they are all voiced, alveolar consonants, you are correct.

The reason it is important to view the classification of consonants in a multidimensional way is it is often essential in assessing and describing disordered sound systems. As creative learners of a sound system, children might develop unique and often idiosyncratic phonological rules that are more complicated and challenging to identify and describe than the single replacement of all fricatives with stops, or "stopping." A child might develop a phonological strategy to accommodate for a limited sound system by producing target voiceless obstruents with [t], as described previously under "Characteristics of a Speech Disorder." Specifically, the child produces [t] for targets /t, k, tʃ, s, ʃ/. As illustrated in the group of sounds that the child collapsed to [t], the common aspect was that they were all voiceless and had members from each of the three classes that comprise the group of sounds called obstruents; for example, stops, affricates, and fricatives. This mistake is not an uncommon phonological error for children who have moderate-to-severe speech disorders. More will be said about phonological errors later in this chapter. Interestingly, the child's error of [t] was also a voiceless obstruent that was produced for the larger class of voiceless obstruents that the child was unable to produce. As discussed previously, this situation is characteristic of a functional speech disorder in which there is a relationship between the phonetic properties of the collapsed adult targets and the child's errored substitution.

You might have noticed that sounds have been listed throughout this section in a particular order: first, within their manner class, and then according to place of production, going from the most anterior to the most posterior place of production. It will be helpful to use this organization in listing a child's sound inventory or phoneme collapse. It is easier to identify any patterns or rules that might exist in a child's system when you use this organization. An illustration of this procedure is demonstrated by a simple listing of a child's phonetic inventory:

[m, z, d, b, w, n, t, p, h]

Looking at the list of sounds produced by the child, we see that it is not immediately obvious how the child's phonetic inventory can be described according to the general characteristics of place, voice, and manner.

Now, notice how much easier it would be to describe the child's phonetic inventory from the following organization of his sounds:

Stops	p b	t d
Nasals	m	n
Glides	w	h
Fricatives	z	

From this organization of the child's phonetic inventory, it is easy to describe the child's inventory as being limited to generally voiced anterior consonants from primarily the classes of stops, nasals, and glides.

Again, knowing the classification of the consonants facilitates your ability to use such an organizational approach to listing phonetic inventories or diagramming phoneme collapses. In turn, the organization facilitates your identification and description of the child's phonological rules.

Consonants: Distinctive Feature Classification

A second way in which consonants can be classified is by distinctive features. Based on distinctive feature theory, phonemes are comprised of a bundle of features that make them distinct from any other phoneme. Distinctive features are binary with a "+" or "–" used to denote the presence or absence of that feature in a particular phoneme. Each distinctive feature typically represents some physiological aspect of sound production. For example, the feature [voice] represents the presence or absence of vocal fold vibration as [+voice] or [–voice], respectively.

To illustrate the binary nature of distinctive features, Figure 1–1 represents a tree diagram of some of the basic distinctive features that could be used to classify the English consonants into their natural classes of nasals, glides, liquids, stops, fricatives, and affricates.

At the top of the diagram is the feature [sonorant]. This feature represents how sounds are produced with regard to openness of the vocal tract and spontaneous voicing. This situation might already sound familiar from the previous discussion under traditional classification of consonants. Those sounds produced with little or no obstruction and with spontaneous voicing would be categorized as [+sonorant] and include nasals, liquids, and glides. Sounds that are produced with partial or complete obstruction in the vocal tract and with or without voicing are classified as [–sonorant]. The feature [sonorant] is a major class feature in that it divides the English consonants into two major classes of sounds: sonorants and obstruents.

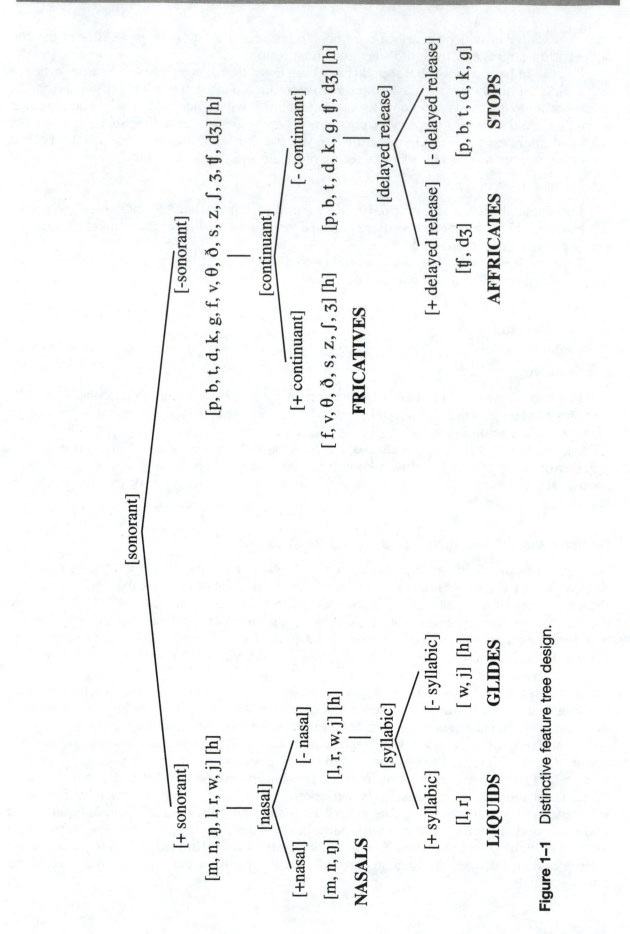

Figure 1–1   Distinctive feature tree design.

Let's stay on the [+sonorant] side and specify the distinctive features needed to classify the sonorants into their natural classes of sounds. One feature that will separate these sounds is the feature [nasal]. Using the binary classification, [+nasal] will describe the nasals separately from the remaining sounds, which are [–nasal]. We still need another distinctive feature to tease out the glides from the liquids. Recall from the previous traditional classifications that liquids can function as either consonants or vowels. The distinctive feature [syllabic] will capture that characteristic of liquids. Thus, [+syllabic] specifies the class of liquids while [–syllabic] describes the glides.

Looking at the left side of our tree diagram, we can see that we have described three of the six natural classes of English consonants (nasals, liquids, and glides) with the features [sonorant, nasal, and syllabic]. To describe the class of liquids, then, we could use the following features:

$$\begin{bmatrix} +\text{sonorant} \\ -\text{nasal} \\ +\text{syllabic} \end{bmatrix}$$

Obviously, this method is a broad way to classify the natural classes of sounds, but hopefully it provides a general idea of how distinctive features are used to classify sounds. Notice that the sounds are described similarly to the traditional classification system, but use the different terminology of distinctive features. As in the traditional classification system, the more features you use, the smaller the class of sounds you will describe until you list all the features that will describe only one sound.

Now, let's move to the right side of the diagram and separate those sounds into their natural classes. A feature that will break this group of sounds apart is the feature [continuant]. Sounds that are [+continuant] include the class of fricatives. Stops and affricates are classified as [–continuant] due to their complete blockage of the airstream.

To separate stops from affricates, the feature [delayed release] can be used. Recall that affricates are produced by a complete blockage and then gradual release of the airstream. Thus, affricates are [+delayed release] and stops are [–delayed release].

We've now described the six natural classes of English consonants using distinctive features. As with the sonorants, we can describe one of the obstruent classes of sounds as a compilation of distinctive features. For example, affricates would be described as follows:

$$\begin{bmatrix} -\text{sonorant} \\ -\text{continuant} \\ +\text{delayed release} \end{bmatrix}$$

We could further describe the obstruent classes with regard to voicing by using the distinctive feature [voice]. To specify a specific sound within a class, additional features would be used. For example, the phoneme /s/ would be described by the following features:

$$\begin{bmatrix} -\text{sonorant} \\ +\text{continuant} \\ -\text{voice} \\ +\text{anterior} \\ +\text{strident} \end{bmatrix}$$

There are several different distinctive feature classifications, but the one most commonly used is by Chomsky and Halle (1968). You will note that several additional distinctive features are used to classify the consonants. In general, each distinctive feature relates to one of the three broad parameters of consonant production involving place, voice, or manner. The correspondence between the distinctive features and the traditional description of place, voice, and manner is provided in Table 1–3.

TABLE 1–3   Correspondence Between PVM and Distinctive Features

Distinctive Feature	Place	Voice	Manner
Sonorant			X
Continuant			X
Nasal			X
Syllabic			X
Consonantal			X
Delayed release			X
Strident	X		X
Anterior	X		
Coronal	X		
Voice		X	

Vowels: Traditional Classification

A traditional classification of the English vowels includes the following descriptions: (1) tongue height; (2) tongue advancement; (3) lip rounding; and (4) tension. Tongue height refers to the vertical placement of the tongue whereas tongue advancement refers to the horizontal placement of the tongue. Lip rounding describes the lips as rounded or unround in the production of vowels. Finally, tension refers to the amount of muscle activity involved in vowel production as either tense or lax. These four parameters of English vowel production are summarized in Table 1–4.

Tongue height (vertical) describes the vowel production with reference to three positions of the tongue: high, mid, or low.

1. high vowels—vowels that are produced with the tongue in its highest position [i, ɪ, u, ʊ]. The mouth is in an almost closed position.

2. mid vowels—vowels that are produced with the tongue in midline position, and the mouth opening is slightly larger [e, ɛ, ʌ, ə, ɚ, ɝ, ɔ, o]

3. low vowels—vowels that are produced with the tongue in its lowest position, and the mouth opening is wide [æ, ɑ]

TABLE 1–4

	Front	Central	Back
High	i ɪ		u ʊ
Mid	e ɛ	ə ɚ ɜˡ	o ɔ
Low	æ	ʌ	ɑ

Tongue advancement (horizontal) describes vowel production with reference to three positions of the tongue: front, central, or back (Table 1–5).

TABLE 1–5

Unrounded Vowels	Neutral Lip-Rounding	Rounded Vowels
[i, ɪ, e, ɛ, æ]	[ʌ, ə, 3ˡ, ɚ]	[u, ʊ, o, ɔ, ɑ]
Front Vowels	Central Vowels	Back Vowels

1. front vowels—vowels that are produced with the tongue in the front of the mouth with a smaller resonating cavity space in the front of the back and larger resonating cavity space in the back of the mouth [i, ɪ, e, ɛ, æ].

2. central vowels—vowels that are produced with the tongue in the central part of the mouth with equal space in front and back of the tongue [ʌ, ə, 3ˡ, ɚ].

3. back vowels—vowels that are produced with the tongue in the back of the mouth with a larger resonating cavity space in the front and a smaller resonating cavity space in the back of the mouth [u, ʊ, o, ɔ, ɑ].

Lip-rounding describes the roundness or retraction of the lips in producing vowels. All back vowels are rounded while all front vowels are unrounded. Central vowels are neutral in lip rounding. This process is intuitively logical, because as the tongue moves posteriorly, the lips protrude. Thus, as the tongue moves from front to central to back vowels, the lips go from unrounded to neutral in lip rounding and finally are rounded.

Tension describes the degree of relative muscle activity involved in vowel production as well as the duration of the vowel. Tense vowels have increased muscle activity and are longer in duration than lax vowels. Tension distinguishes between vowels that are the same height and advancement. For example, [i, ɪ] are both front, high vowels. They are distinguished, however, by tension in that [i] is tense and [ɪ] is lax. Further, all stressed vowels, such as [ʌ, 3ˡ], are tense vowels. Conversely, the unstressed vowels [ə, ɚ] are lax (Table 1–6).

These four parameters of vowel production (tongue height, tongue advancement, lip rounding, and tension) can be combined to describe a single vowel. For example, back, high, tense, and round describes the vowel [u].

TABLE 1–6

	Tense Vowels	Lax Vowels
Front	[i, e]	[ɪ, ɛ, æ]
Central	[ʌ, ɝ]	[ə, ɚ]
Back	[u, o]	[ʊ, ɔ, ɑ]

ɝ, ɚ

Similar to having a multidimensional understanding of the place, voice, and manner classification of consonants, it is important to have the same thorough understanding of vowel classification. Again, the reason is due to an accurate description and analysis of the child's sound system. Many phonological rules are formulated on the basis of the following vowel. Several studies have been reported (cf., Camarata and Gandour, 1984; Williams and Dinnsen, 1987) in which the vowel environment conditioned the occurrence of a particular consonant. A specific example of the importance of accurate vowel transcription and knowledge of vowel classification was reported by Williams and Dinnsen (1987). In this case study of a child (NE age 4 years, 6 months) with a severe functional speech disorder, a phonological process analysis of the child's speech revealed several inconsistent error patterns, as shown in Table 1–7.

TABLE 1–7

Fronting	Backing	Velar Assimilation
[te] "cage" BUT: [ko] "comb"	[kɑ] "Tom" BUT: [di] "teeth"	[gɑ] "dog" BUT: [dɛ] "leg"
[deʔ] "gate" BUT: [goʔ] "goat"	[guʰ] "tooth" BUT: [dɛ] "dress"	

By ignoring the influence of the following vowel, an inaccurate description and analysis of NE's speech was obtained. In this incorrect analysis, three different phonological processes were identified, and each was used inconsistently. Not only was there little descriptive or explanatory information provided by this analysis, but there is also no informed direction for intervention.

If, however, the vowel environment is examined, then NE's error pattern becomes apparent. Notice that NE produced alveolar stops before front vowels and velar stops before back vowels. What was originally described as an inconsistent application of three different processes can now be consistently described by one rule. Furthermore, the rule is explanatory in terms of assimilation: front consonants are produced in the environment of front vowels while back consonants are produced in the environment of back vowels. The rule is consistent, logical, and even predictable. Finally, knowing that the vowel environment conditioned the preceding consonant, the SLP can make an informed clinical decision regarding intervention. Specifically, the SLP would know that NE does not need to learn to produce alveolar or velar stops but that he needs to learn to produce them across different vowel environments. The SLP needs to design an intervention program that will teach NE to produce velars before front vowels and alveolars before back vowels.

This section is a rather lengthy discussion to point out the importance of accurate vowel transcription and knowledge of vowel classification. Demonstrating the clinical application of such knowledge and its impact on clinical diagnosis and treatment, however, hopefully highlights the significance and usefulness of this knowledge.

Vowels: Distinctive Feature Classification

As with the consonants, vowels can also be classified by using distinctive features. Vowels are described primarily by the features [low], [high], [back], [round], and [tense] in addition to some of the previously described features of [sonorant], [syllabic], and [consonantal].

First, all vowels are [+sonorant] because the vocal tract is relatively open and there is spontaneous voicing. Vowels are also [+syllabic] because they can form a syllable. Because vowels are not consonants, they are [–consonantal]. Thus, the feature matrix for vowels would be:

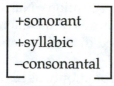

$$\begin{bmatrix} +\text{sonorant} \\ +\text{syllabic} \\ -\text{consonantal} \end{bmatrix}$$

To specify a certain class of vowels, such as high vowels or front vowels or even a specific vowel, additional features needed to be added to this feature matrix. That is where the new features of [low], [high], [back], and [tense] are used. The features [low] and [high] are used to describe the vertical movement of the tongue, or tongue height. These features are described as follows for high, mid, and low vowels:

high vowels	[+high]
mid vowels	$\begin{bmatrix} -\text{high} \\ -\text{low} \end{bmatrix}$
low vowels	[+low]

The features [back] and [round] are used to describe the horizontal placement of the tongue, or tongue advancement. Front, central, and back vowels are described by these features:

front vowels	[–back]
central vowels	$\begin{bmatrix} +\text{back} \\ -\text{round} \end{bmatrix}$
back vowels	[+back]

Notice that the feature [round] was not needed to describe front or back vowels. Recall that in English, all front vowels are unround and all back vowels are rounded. Thus, it is redundant to add [–round] to front vowels that are [–back] or to add [+round] to back vowels that are [+back]. This feature is only necessary to distinguish central from back vowels.

Finally, the feature [tense] distinguishes between vowels at the same height and advancement. For example, the vowel [ɪ] would be described by the following feature matrix:

$$\left[\begin{array}{l} +\text{sonorant} \\ +\text{syllabic} \\ -\text{consonantal} \\ +\text{high} \\ -\text{back} \\ +\text{tense} \end{array}\right]$$

As with the consonants, distinctive features correspond with the traditional classification of tongue height, tongue advancement, lip rounding, and tension in describing the English vowels.

Diacritic Symbols

So far, the discussion of phonetic transcription has focused on broad transcription. Narrow phonetic transcription is often needed, however, to capture important features of the client's productions by using diacritic symbols. Shriberg and Kent (1995) described diacritic symbols according to eight primary categories that include symbols for stress, nasal, lip, tongue, sound source, stop release, timing, and juncture. Examples of some of the more commonly used diacritics in clinical phonetics are listed in Table 1–8. For a complete list of diacritic symbols and categories, readers are referred to Shriberg and Kent (1995).

TABLE 1–8

Category	Diacritic Symbol	
Nasal Symbols	Nasalized	~
	Nasal emission	÷
	Denasalized	⊬
Lip Symbols	Labialized (rounded) consonant	ω
	Nonlabialized (unrounded) consonant	ω
Tongue Symbols	Dentalized	˛
	Palatalized	ɹ
	Lateralized	˄
Sound Source Symbols	Partially voiced	v
	Partially devoiced	o
Stop Release Symbols	Aspirated	h
	Unaspirated	=
	Unreleased	˥
Timing Symbols	Lengthened	:

Phonetic Transcription

This section began with phonetic transcription, and we shall end this section with a brief discussion of phonetic transcription. As we stated previously, transcription is the foundation on which everything you will do with children with speech disorders is based. For a more detailed discussion of phonetic transcription of disordered speech, readers are referred to a recent article by Powell (2001). The following is a list of helpful suggestions in phonetically transcribing children's speech:

1. If you feel that your transcription skills are rusty, review the preceding sections, refer to them as a resource as needed, and practice transcribing. Develop your own summary sheets or "cheat sheets" to help you with your transcriptions and classification. Write your grocery lists, the alphabet, days of the week, months of the year, your name, and a note to a friend as ways to practice your transcription. You might even build up to transcribing the reporter on the evening news.

2. Do whole-word transcriptions when administering sound inventory tests with your clients.

3. Do online transcription. Nothing can replace the visual cues and auditory clarity of live transcription.

4. Audio-record the child's responses so that you have a backup to check your transcriptions. Videotaped data can also be used.

5. Purchase a clipboard, which will facilitate your ability to get closer to the client and transcribe more easily.

6. Seat your client in the large adult chair, and you should sit in the small child's seat. This situation will bring the child up and you down so that the child's mouth is more visible, which will facilitate your ability to transcribe the child's productions.

7. Remember to *watch* the child's mouth as he or she produces the words. Then, transcribe what you heard. Often, we're ready to transcribe with our heads down and then miss the visual cues that online transcription provides.

8. Ask the child to repeat as often as necessary to get the best transcription without losing the child's attention or cooperation. If the child becomes agitated by frequent repetitions, explain to the child that you want to be sure to write it down *exactly* as he or she said it, so you might have to ask him or her to repeat a couple of times. It might also help to move on to another item and return to the difficult item later during the test.

9. If you are unsure of how to transcribe a particular sound, write something that is as close to what you hear as possible. For example, if it is a fricative, write "F"; write "V" for vowel, and so on. Then, re-listen to the audio recording to see whether you can determine the appropriate symbol for the sound that was produced.

10. Use pencils with good erasers.

11. Use colleagues for periodic reliability checks.

As may be obvious at this point, nothing can replace good, solid phonetic transcription in establishing an efficacious program of intervention for children with speech disorders. Be patient in developing or re-establishing your phonetic transcription skills. As with other skills, it takes time and practice to become proficient. The reward will be in the payoff of improved diagnoses, easier planning and implementation of the treatment, and decreased treatment time for your client.

NORMAL PHONOLOGICAL DEVELOPMENT

Normal phonological acquisition can be described in terms of four periods of development. These include the prelinguistic period (birth to 1 year), first words (1 year to 1 $1/2$), phonemic development ($1^1/_2$ to 4 years), and stabilization (4 to 8 years). We will briefly describe each of these periods of development in sections that follow.

Prelinguistic Period (*Birth–1 Year*)

In the first period, the prelinguistic period, the infant moves from reflexive vocalizations to adult-like syllables. Oller (1980) described five stages of development within the prelinguistic period: phonation, cooing, expansion, canonical, and variegated babbling stages.

Phonation Stage (Birth–1 Month)

The infant's vocalizations are characterized by a predominance of reflexive vocalizations that include hunger and discomfort cries and vegetative activities (for example, burps, hiccups).

Cooing Stage (2–4 Months)

The infant's cooing and gooing are regular and repetitive with velar sounds, including the back rounded vowel /u/.

Expansion Stage (4–6 Months)

The infant's vocalizations are characterized by several different types of vocalization that include raspberries, squealing, growling, and yelling. This stage has been described as exploratory phonetic behavior. The types of vocalizations can vary from day to day. In this stage, marginal babbling begins to occur.

Canonical Babbling (6–8 Months)

The infant's vocalizations are characterized by the reduplication of syllables, such as ba-ba-ba or ma-ma-ma. There is a lack of variation in that the same consonants are repeated in syllable strings. The syllables are more "speech-like," and the intonation patterns are more adult-like.

Variegated Babbling (9–12 Months)

The infant's vocalizations are similar to the canonical babbling, but they have more variety, such as [bɑwɪdɑ]. This stage is frequently regarded as the onset of "true speech." These vocalizations are also referred to as jargon and are often mistaken for real words by caregivers.

First Words (*12 Months–18 Months*)

During this period of phonological acquisition, lexical development and phonological development are closely intertwined. The child appears to learn and produce new vocabulary words as whole, unanalyzed units rather than as sequences of segments. Early productions, therefore, cannot be described in terms of phonemes because there is not a stable correspondence within and across lexical items. As a consequence of this whole-word strategy in acquiring words, the acquisition of vocabulary is largely driven by the sounds that the child can produce. Specifically, the child actively selects vocabulary that includes sounds that he or she can produce (IN phonology) and avoids words that include sounds that he or she cannot produce (OUT phonology). Schwartz and Leonard (1982) found that children typically used this strategy for consonants that occurred at the beginning of words. This finding is significant because it indicates that the child has the beginnings of an organized phonology because he or she responds differently to sounds already acquired versus those target sounds that are not yet part of his or her phonemic repertoire.

This whole-word strategy works for the young child while the vocabulary is within the 50-word stage. After that point, the strategy is no longer efficient.

The child's speech is characterized by the production of simple syllabic structures (CV, CVC, and CVCV), and their phonetic inventory consists primarily of stops, nasals, and glides. With regard to place of production, labial and alveolar consonants tend to be frequent whereas palatals and velars are less frequent.

Phonemic Period (*18 Months–4 Years*)

The rapid increase in vocabulary that generally occurs after the 50-word stage at the 18-month level forces the child to develop a different strategy in acquiring new lexical items into his or her vocabulary. The child changes from a whole-word approach to rule-governed forms that have a stable, segmental correspondence with the adult words. This change results in a system that is based primarily on phonemes rather than on whole words. Two characteristics of this period of phonological acquisition include:

   a. A rapid increase in vocabulary size and a relaxation of selection constraints on adult words attempted by the child

   b. The relationship between the sounds of the adult model and the child's pronunciation becomes more systematic (rule-governed).

Stabilization Period (*4–8 Years*)

During this period of phonological development, children stabilize their pronunciations of phonemes that had been produced variably and acquire the last phonemes needed for completion of the phonetic inventory. Generally, stops, nasals, and glides are mastered first, followed by liquids and finally fricatives and affricates. Initial consonants are mastered earlier than final consonants, particularly before voiced final consonants. Clusters are typically acquired last.

The stages of normal phonological development are summarized in Table 1–9.

Developmental Norms

At this point, a short discussion about the establishment of age norms for English consonant acquisition seems warranted. A number of studies have been conducted to determine the age at which typically developing children acquire the consonants of the English language. These studies are generally cross-sectional, in which a large number of children at different age levels are tested at a single point in time on their ability to produce speech sounds. The investigators establish criterion levels for determining the age of acquisition for the group as a whole. Different criterion levels have been used that range from a stringent criterion level of 90% accuracy to 75% accuracy and finally to a 50% criterion level that reflects "customary production" rather than "mastery" (Sander, 1972). Another difference across studies is the

TABLE 1–9

Prelinguistic Period (birth–1 year)	First Words (12–18 months)	Phonemic Period (18 months–4 years)	Stabilization Period (4–8 years)
Phonation Stage (birth–1 month): reflexive vocalizations Cooing Stage (2–4 months): cooing/gooing with velar sounds and /u/ Expansion Stage (4–6 months): exploratory vocalizations; for example, raspberries, squeals, growls, and so on. Canonical Babbling (6–8 months): reduplicated syllable strings, such as, ba-ba-ba Variegated Babbling (9–12 months): variety in babbled syllables; often referred to as "jargon"	* First vocabulary words learned as whole, unanalyzed units; therefore, there is no stable correspondence within and across lexical items * Child actively selects and avoids vocabulary that contains sounds that are IN or OUT of their phonetic repertoire * Simple syllable structure with primarily stops, nasals, and glides produced at labial and alveolar places of production	* Rapid increase in vocabulary which forces child to switch from whole-word strategy to rule-based strategy * The relationship between the sounds of the adult model and the child's pronunciation becomes more systematic (rule-governed).	* Pronunciations of phonemes that had been variably produced become stabilized. * The last phonemes are acquired to complete the child's phonetic inventory. * Typically clusters are acquired last.

methodology used to collect the normative data that includes (1) imitation versus spontaneous productions; (2) the number of positions assessed (initial, medial, and final); and (3) reporting "full" versus "partial" data from children.

These differences in criterion levels and methodology are important considerations for SLPs using these norms, because a relative small difference in methodology can result in a great difference in the age of acquisition that the studies report. A final caution in using developmental norms is that recent studies of small groups of children have found that individual differences across children are so great that it might be impossible to establish meaningful age norms. Given these cautions, it is not possible to determine an exact age in which a given sound can be expected to be produced correctly. Rather, it is better to use norms as a general picture of acquisition.

With these cautions in mind, Table 1–10 summarizes the age norms across three different studies that utilized three different criterion levels (50%, 75%, and 90%). You will notice many similarities across studies, but there are also differences observed across studies and across criterion levels.

TABLE 1–10   Normative Acquisition of English Consonants According to Three Studies (50%, 75%, and 90% Criterion Levels)

Consonant	Prather, Hedrick, and Kern (1975)		Sander (1972)		Smit et al. (1990)	
	50%	90%	50%	90%	50%	75%
n	< 24	24	< 24	36	< 36	<36
m	< 24	24	< 24	36	< 36	<36
p	< 24	24	< 24	36	< 36	<36
h	< 24	24	< 24	36	< 36	<90
t	< 24	32	24	<48	< 36	<36
k	24	32	24	44	< 36	<36
f	< 24	36	32	48	< 36	42
w	< 24	40	< 24	40	< 36	<36
ŋ	< 24	36	24	>48	< 36	<90
b	24	36	< 24	48	< 36	<36
g	24	36	24	48	< 36	<36
s	24	44	36	>48	42	60
j	28	32	30	48	< 36	42
d	28	36	24	48	< 36	<36
ʍ	28	>48	Not assessed		Not assessed	
l	32	>48	36	>48	42	72
r	32	>48	36	>48	42	72
ʃ	36	>48	42	>48	42	60
tʃ	36	>48	42	>48	42	72
dʒ	36	>48	48	>48	42	54
v	40	>48	48	>48	42	54
z	44	>48	42	>48	48	72
ʒ	44	>48	44	>48	Not assessed	
ð	48	>48	48	>48	54	66
θ	48	>48	48	>48	54	72

The data source for these norms are Prather, Hedrick, and Kern (1975); Sander (1972); and Smit, Hand, Frelinger, Bernthal, and Byrd (1990).

ASSESSING PRE-LINGUISTIC AND EARLY LINGUISTIC VOCALIZATIONS

With the federal legislation of PL 99-457 that mandates the provision of early identification and intervention for children from birth to 3 years of age, SLPs are seeing younger children in their caseloads. The procedures for assessing the pre-linguistic and early linguistic vocalizations are different than those used with older children. Rather than using a standard sound inventory test like those used with many older children, the SLP must incorporate different sampling procedures. Specifically, Stoel-Gammon (1987) recommended using two sampling procedures with young children (Table 1–11). One sampling procedure is an unstructured sample of the child's speech during free play, preferably with a caregiver. Based on information we have about phonological acquisition, children at these earlier ages tend to actively select and avoid words that contain sounds that are IN or OUT of their phonetic inventories. Therefore, it is important to supplement this unstructured sample with an elicited sample in order to provide the child opportunities to produce words that contain a representative sampling of the English sounds at least in word-initial and word-final positions. Using real objects is easier for eliciting responses from younger children than the pictured objects that are frequently used in the sound inventory tests for older children. The SLP can develop his or her own list of words and set of objects for assessing young children or use the list of words that were developed to sample all English sounds at least once in every word position. This list is included in Appendix A.

TABLE 1–11

Two Types of Speech Samples

- Unstructured, free play with caregiver

- Elicited, single words representing all English sounds at least in word-initial and word-final positions using real objects (see Appendix A)

After the samples of the child's speech have been collected, how does the SLP analyze them? Again, these children are at an earlier stage of phonological development, and the rule-based analyses might not be appropriate to describe their sound systems at this point. Many of these children are in the first words stage and have fewer than 50 words in their lexicon. Based largely on the work by Stoel-Gammon (1985, 1987), Williams and Elbert (2002) utilized both independent and relational analyses to describe early sound systems (Table 1–12). Independent analyses describe the child's sound system as a unique, self-contained system separate from the adult or target sound system. The child's phonetic inventory and syllable structure are described without judgment of accuracy or reference to the adult system. Relational analyses are what SLPs typically use when describing children's sound systems. This type of analysis describes the child's system *in relation* to the adult system in terms of accuracy. Relational analyses can include Percent Consonants Correct (PCC; Shriberg and Kwiatkowski, 1982) as well as pattern analyses that describe the child's error patterns in terms of place-voice-manner or phonological processes.

Stoel-Gammon and others suggest that only meaningful utterances are analyzed for children in the first words stage. For pre-linguistic children, their vocalizations can be analyzed according to *Mean Babbling Level* (MBL) described by Stoel-Gammon (1989), vocalization rate (Rescorla and Ratner, 1996), sound preferences, and syllable structure.

TABLE 1–12

Independent and Relational Analyses

- Independent Analyses—describes the child's sound system as a unique, self-contained system independent of the adult sound system; generally includes a description of the child's phonetic inventory and syllable structure

- Relational Analyses—describes the child's sound system *in relation* to the adult system in terms of accuracy of sound productions; can describe errors in terms of substitutions, omissions, distortions, or additions (SODA) or in terms of error patterns, such as place-voice-manner or phonological processes

Late Talkers: Delay Versus Deviance

Most of the normative data available to SLPs addresses the phonological development of older children, ages 3 to 8. Recently, however, several studies have contributed to an expanded database for the development of children under 3 years of age. In addition, recent investigations have attempted to identify potential predictor variables that might help distinguish at an earlier age those children who will "outgrow" their delay from children who will require direct intervention in order to "catch up" with their age peers (cf., Paul and Jennings, 1992; Rescorla and Ratner, 1996; Stoel-Gammon, 1991; Williams and Elbert, 2002).

Stoel-Gammon (1991) described several potential "red flags" in phonological development that might signal normal from disordered phonological development (Table 1–13). At 24 months of age, these included numerous vowel errors, widespread deletion of initial consonants, substitution of glottal consonants or [h] for a variety of consonants, substitution of back consonants for front consonants, and the deletion of final consonants.

TABLE 1–13

"Red Flags" in Early Phonological Development (Stoel-Gammon, 1991)

- numerous vowel errors

- deletion of initial consonants

- substitution of glottal consonants or [h] for a variety of consonants

- substitution of back consonants for front consonants

- deletion of final consonants

Williams and Elbert (2002) followed five late talkers for monthly observations over the course of a year to examine any potential differences between children who "outgrew" their speech delay versus those children who did not. The children were grouped into a younger group (22–33 months) and an older group (31– 41 months). Based on their results, variables that appeared to be the most predictive of the late talkers' phonological skills at 33 months included sound variability, syllable diversity, atypical error patterns, and rate of resolution.

Specifically, those children who did not "catch up" with their age peers by the end of the study exhibited greater sound variability, which appeared to reflect an immature and less stable sound system; they produced primarily simple syllable structures with little diversity; their errors were more idiosyncratic and atypical and often involved early as well as later developing sounds; and finally, little or no change was noted for the children whose phonological development was characterized as deviant across all domains of phonological development (in other words, phonetic inventory, syllable structure, syllable diversity or complexity; PCC, and phonological variability) (Table 1–14). It should be noted that children who did not "catch up" were in the older group and had more limited inventories, less diversity, and greater variation than the younger group even at an older age. It is important to note that the two children who did not evidence spontaneous remission were not identified as late talkers until age 30 and 31 months. Rescorla and Schwartz (1990) suggested that the likelihood of a child outgrowing his or her delay decreases if the child is 30 months old when first diagnosed with a delay.

TABLE 1–14

Delayed Phonological Development	*Deviant Phonological Development*
Larger phonetic inventories • 13–15 word-initial (WI) consonants; 8–11 word-final (WF) consonants at 32 months	Severely limited phonetic inventories • 6–9 WI consonants; 1–5 WF consonants at 32 months
Greater diversity in syllable structures • mean of 9.2 different syllables from age 22–33 months	Limited diversity in syllable structures • mean of 7.5 different syllable structures from 30–41 months
More complex syllable structures • mean of 5.4 complex syllables from age 22–33 months	Simple syllable structures • mean of 1.1. complex syllables from age 30–41 months
Higher PCC • mean PCC of .56 for 31–33 months	Lower PCC • mean PCC of .34 for 40–41 months
Lower sound variability • mean variability of 1.2 for 31–33 months	Greater sound variability • mean variability of 1.74 for 40–41 months
Typical error patterns	Atypical error patterns
Rate of resolution: consistent and steady	Rate of resolution: little or no change

SECTION

ASSESSMENT PROCEDURES

● ●

This section includes information on standardized and non-standardized assessment procedures of children's sound systems. Each topic will be addressed with answers to the following questions:

WHO?	Specifies the population for whom the topic applies; generally children with functional speech disorders
WHAT?	Specifies the topic, such as independent analysis
WHY?	Specifies the rationale or importance of the topic (for example, to adequately describe the child's sound system)
HOW?	Lists specific procedures in which the topic can be completed

Research Support

When appropriate, results from research studies will be provided to support a particular topic.

VARIABLES TO CONSIDER IN ASSESSMENT OF CHILD SPEECH DISORDERS

WHO?	SLPs completing an assessment of children's speech
WHAT?	Variables that must be considered in assessing children's speech
WHY?	To obtain appropriate and adequate data for the assessment of children's speech
HOW?	Determining the best methods to collect assessment data considering important client variables

- Age of child (some procedures, as discussed in following sections, are more appropriate for younger children [12–36 months] than for older children [preschool to school-age])
- Severity of speech disorder (more severe disorders might require more extensive single-word testing than is possible with a published sound inventory test)
- Type of test (sound inventory, pattern test, conversational sample)
- Length of sample (sound inventory tests are generally short and range from 35–60 items; some tests recommend a minimum of 100–250 words from a conversational sample; still others (for example, Gierut's Productive Phonological Knowledge Protocol) use a 196-item single-word protocol to elicit specific types of productions in order to assess the child's productive phonological knowledge)
- Recording of child's responses (different options are available, including simple plus/minus scoring or single phone transcription; however, whole-word transcription is strongly recommended [see the section on "Phonetic Transcription"])

SPEECH SAMPLING

WHO?	Children (infants to school-age) with suspected speech disorders
WHAT?	Sampling procedures to assess speech and phonological skills
WHY?	To assess the speech abilities of children
HOW?	Collecting single word and connected speech samples in order to obtain the most representative speech sample

- As we discussed under "Variables in Assessment of Child Speech," different sampling procedures are available to assess a child's speech.
- Single-word elicited samples (sound inventory standardized or non-standardized instruments) are most commonly used to assess children's speech.
- Conversational speech is frequently recommended to supplement single-word productions in order to compare the child's intelligibility in both contexts.
  - Some recommended sampling procedures for connected speech include:
    - Story-retelling
    - Story generation
    - Expository speech

- Interaction during free or unstructured play
- Reading (for school-age children)

SPEECH SCREENING

WHO?	Children (generally toddlers to school-age)
WHAT?	Screening of articulatory skills
WHY?	To determine whether speech development is normal and whether further in-depth testing is required
HOW?	Using standardized and non-standardized instruments

- Non-standardized and standardized instruments can be used to screen a child's speech. Either type of test should be able to be administered in a relatively short time period (about five minutes).
- Non-standardized tests can include asking the child to answer simple questions (such as, "What is your name?", "What is your favorite toy/game/movie?", and "What did you do today?"), repeat a short list of words that sample early, mid, and later-developing phonemes, recite the alphabet, the days of the week, and count (if appropriate).
- Standardized tests are also available and include the following:
  - *Preschool Language Scale 3 (PLS-3)* by Zimmerman, Steiner, and Pond (1992)
  - *Quick Screen of Phonology (QSP)* by Bankson and Bernthal (1990)
  - *Speech and Language Screening Test for Preschool Children* (also known as the Fluharty) by Fluharty (1978)
  - *Templin-Darley Screening Test* (in the *Templin-Darley Tests of Articulation*) by Templin and Darley (1969)
  - *Joliet 3-Minute Preschool Speech and Language Screen* by Kinzler (1992)
  - *Joliet 3-Minute Speech and Language Screen (Revised)* by Kinzler and Johnson (1992)
  - *Screening Speech Articulation Test* by Mecham, Jex, and Jones (1970)
  - *Watts Articulation Test for Screening (WATS)* by Watts and Paynter (1973)

WORD PROBES OR DEEP TESTING

WHO?	Children with speech disorders (generally toddler to school-age)
WHAT?	Word probes that sample the child's productions of specific sounds in greater depth
WHY?	(1) To provide information regarding the consistency of child's productions, (2) To identify possible facilitating contexts, (3) To determine clinical goals
HOW?	Elicit target sound(s) in multiple and diverse exemplars

- It is frequently difficult to determine the consistency of a child's error productions on the basis of a sound inventory test or to identify phonetic contexts in which the child's production might be correct. In these situations, more in-depth testing might be required or desired by the SLP.
- Different word lists or tests are available to "deep test" a particular sound or error pattern.
  - Bleile (1995) provides several "Word Probes for Error Patterns" that include probes for error patterns involving changes in place of production, manner of production, voicing, deletion, and reduplication.
  - Clinical Probes of Articulation Consistency (C-PAC) by Secord (1981)
  - McDonald Deep Test of Articulation
  - Contextual Test of Articulation (CTA) by Aase, Hovre, Krause, Schelfhout, Smith, and Carpenter (2000)
- SLPs can choose to "deep test" a sound or error pattern in order to determine the consistency of the error and to identify possible phonetic contexts in which the sound is produced correctly. This information is frequently used in intervention planning.
- Specifically, inconsistent errors can be selected on the premise that variability might be an important indicator of flexibility and change. For a different perspective, however, see research support on consistency of error patterns in intervention outcomes.
- In traditional methods of speech intervention, SLPs planned intervention on target sounds in phonetic contexts in which the child was successful. This approach reflects an articulatory perspective that is not necessarily used as the basis for phonologic intervention planning.

Research Support

Forrest, Elbert, and Dinnsen (2000) found that children who received intervention on a consistent substitute error sound learned the treated sound and generalized it to other contexts. Conversely, children who received intervention on a variable substitute sound did not learn the treated sound. They concluded that substitution variability has a critical impact on treatment outcomes.

COMPONENTS OF A SPEECH ASSESSMENT BATTERY
(INFANT–TODDLER)

WHO?	Children with functional speech disorders (12 months to 3 years)
WHAT?	Assessment battery
WHY?	To provide a thorough assessment of a young child's speech in order to determine speech delay or deviant phonological development
HOW?	Generally through a one to two-hour diagnostic session

- Case history information from the parent(s) or guardian(s)

- Parent questionnaires are very useful for this age group, including *The MacArthur Communicative Development Inventories* (*CDI*; Fenson, Dale, Reznick, Thal, Bates, Hartung, Pethick, and Reilly, 1993) and *Vineland Adaptive Behavior Scales* (Sparrow, Balla, and Cicchetti, 1984)

- Hearing screening (for example, sound field or visually reinforced audiometry [VRA])

- Oral-mechanism evaluation or cursory oral examination (for example, *Oral Speech Mechanism Screening Examination-Third Edition* (*OSMSE-3*) by St. Louis and Ruscello (1987).

- Free play with caretaker using manipulative toys and age-appropriate books to elicit a spontaneous language sample. The sample will be analyzed for lexicon size, type/token ratio, MLU, and semantic relations expressed by using 1–2 word utterances.

- Single-word elicited speech using toys and objects that represent all English sounds, at least in the word-initial and word-final positions (see Appendix A for a sample list)

- Sound play and sound imitation, particularly for younger children (for example, animal sounds, raspberries, clicks, and so on)

- Songs, such as "Old McDonald Had a Farm," "Pop Goes the Weasel," "Eensy, Wensy Spider," "If You're Happy and You Know It," and so on

- Receptive language testing (for example, *Preschool Language Scale-3* (*PLS-3*) by Zimmerman, 1992; *Sequenced Inventory of Communicative Development-Revised* (*SICD-R*) by Hedrick, Prather, and Tobin, 1984)

- Along with receptive language assessment, informal assessment of the child's ability to follow simple commands using an array of real objects for one-step, two-step, and three-step commands. See Appendix B for an example of an informal assessment of commands.

- Assessment of play behavior using informal methods or play assessment instruments. See Tables 2–1 and 2–2 for a description of symbolic play development (adapted from McCune-Nicolich and Carroll, 1981) and some play assessment instruments.

- A summary of an assessment battery for infants and toddlers is organized in Table 2–3.

TABLE 2–1

Stage	Age	Play Behaviors
Pre-symbolic	10–11 months	Pre-play/pre-symbolic schemes • Understands functions of objects
Centered Symbolic	12 months	Autosymbolic • Common actions enacted by child with self
Decentered Symbolic	15 months	Single-scheme symbolic • Applies actions to others (decentered play)

(continues)

TABLE 2–1 *(continued)*

Stage	Age	Play Behaviors
Symbolic Combinations	18 months	Combinatorial symbolic games • Child joins two or more pretend behaviors in a sequence. There are two types of sequences: (1) Applies same sequence to multiple participants (for example, feeds mother, doll, and self) (2) Applies different schemes to one participant (for example, feeds doll, puts to bed, covers with blanket)
Hierarchial Symbolic Combinations	24 months	Hierarchial symbolic combinations • Child plans game or pretend actions prior to performing them
Sociodramatic Play	3–5 years	Pretend games with two or more children • Role assignments (for example, mother, baby, doctor) • Negotiating roles and rules of game • Play structure has a beginning, middle, and end

TABLE 2–2

Play Assessment Instrument	Description
Play Assessment Scale (Fewell and Vadasy, 1984)	The child interacts with a specified set of toys. Play sequences are noted on the scale, which provides a play age.
The Symbolic Play Test (Lowe and Costello, 1976)	The child's spontaneous play is evaluated by using four specified sets of miniature objects.
A Manual for Analyzing Free Play (McCune-Nicholich, 1980)	The child's symbolic play is analyzed according to Piagetian stages by using an organized format with a specified set of toys.
Symbolic Play Checklist (Westby, 1980)	Symbolic play is assessed as part of an integrated component of language, cognitive, and social skills by using a 10-step hierarchy. It can be used for children ages 9 months to 5 years.

TABLE 2–3

Background Information	Speech	Receptive Language	Expressive Language	Play	Other
Case history form	Single-word elicited sample using toys and objects that represent all English sounds, at least in the WI and WF positions (see Appendix A)	Standardized tests, for example, *PLS-3* or *SICD-R*	Standardized tests, for example, *PLS-3* or *SICD-R*	Play assessment instruments (see Table 2–2)	Hearing screening by using sound field or VRA
Parent questionnaire (for example, CDI and Vineland)	Free play sample with caregiver using manipulative toys and age-appropriate books	Informal measures, for example, ability to follow commands (see Appendix B)	Free play sample to assess lexicon, semantic relations, and type/token ratio	Informal play assessment (see development of symbolic play)	Oral mechanism examination
	Sound play and sound imitation				
	Songs				

COMPONENTS OF A SPEECH ASSESSMENT BATTERY (PRESCHOOL TO SCHOOL-AGE)

WHO?	Children with functional speech disorders (preschool to school-age)
WHAT?	Assessment battery
WHY?	To provide a thorough assessment of the child's speech and any potential etiological factors related to the speech disorder
HOW?	Generally through a one to two-hour diagnostic session

- Case history information from the parent(s) or guardian(s)
- Pertinent medical, educational, and/or psychological reports
- Hearing screening and tympanometry
- Oral-mechanism evaluation (for example, *Oral Speech Mechanism Screening Examination-Third Edition* (*OSMSE-3*; St. Louis and Ruscello, 1987)
- Single-word elicited test or sound inventory test (for example, *Goldman-Fristoe Test of Articulation-2* by Goldman and Fristoe, 1999); see Tables 2–5 through 2–8 for additional

published tests. Non-standardized speech test instruments can also be administered to elicit more in-depth samples of the child's speech (see the section on non-standardized speech test instruments)

- Stimulability testing (see the stimulability section)
- Conversational speech sample (to evaluate intelligibility in connected speech as well as to compare single-word productions to connected speech; also to evaluate expressive language skills)
- Phonological awareness testing (for example, *Phonological Awareness Test* by Robertson and Salter, 1997 or *Comprehensive Test of Phonological Processing* (CTOPP; Wagner, Torgesen, and Rashotte, 1999)
- Language testing (for example, *Peabody-Picture Vocabulary Test-III* by Dunn and Dunn, 1997; *Test of Language Development-Primary: 3* by Newcomer and Hammill, 1997)
- A summary of an assessment battery for preschool to school-age children is organized in Table 2–4.

TABLE 2–4

Background Information	Speech	Receptive Language	Expressive Language	Other
Case history	Single-word elicited sample, (for example, GFTA-2) or non-standardized speech test instruments (for example, PKP or SPP)	Standardized tests, for example, PPVT-III, TOLD-P:3	Standardized tests, for example, TOLD-P:3	Hearing screening and tympanometry
Pertinent medical, educational, or psychological reports	Conversational speech sample to assess intelligibility		Language sample to assess morphosyntax and discourse skills	Oral mechanism examination (for example, OSMSE-3)
	Stimulability testing			Phonological awareness testing (for example, PAT or C-TOPP)

PUBLISHED TEST INSTRUMENTS (SOUND INVENTORY TESTS)

WHO?	Children with speech disorders (generally preschool to school-age)
WHAT?	Published sound inventory tests
WHY?	To assess the articulatory skills of preschool to school-age children
HOW?	Administer standardized tests according to the individual test's instructions

- See Table 2–5 for a list of published sound inventory tests that includes information regarding (1) the type of sample, (2) the sample size, and (3) the appropriate ages.

TABLE 2–5 List of Published Sound Inventory Tests

Tests	Type of Sample	Sample Size	Appropriate Ages
ALPHA (Assessment Link Between Phonology and Articulation) Phonology Test-Revised, Robert J. Lowe, 1995; ALPHA Speech & Language Resources	delayed sentence imitation	50 target words embedded in short sentences	3–8 years
Fisher-Logemann Test of Articulation Competence, Hilda Fisher and Jeri Logemann, 1971; Pro-Ed	word and sentence	15 sentences 109 words	3–80+ years
Arizona Articulation Proficiency Scale-2nd Edition (AAPA-2), Janet Fudala and William Reynolds, 1986; Western Psychological Services	words	48 words 25 sentences	1.6–13.11 years
Goldman-Fristoe Test of Articulation-2 (GFTA-2), Ronald Goldman and Macalyne Fristoe, 1999; AGS	words/sentences	35 words 9 sentences	2–16+ years
Photo Articulation Test-2nd Edition (PAT-2), Kathleen Pendergast, Stanley Dickey, John Selma, and Anton Soder, 1984; Pro-Ed.	words	75 words	3.6–8 years
Templin-Darley Test of Articulation, Mildred Templin and Fredic Darley, 1969; Speech Bin	words/sentences	141 words	3–8 years

(continues)

TABLE 2–5   *(continued)*

Tests	Type of Sample	Sample Size	Appropriate Ages
Test of Minimal Articulation Competence (T-MAC), Wayne Secord, 1981; Psychological Corporation	words	107 items	3–80+ years
Weiss Comprehensive Articulation Test (WCAT), Curtis Weiss, 1980; Pro-Ed	words	50 words	preschool–adult

PUBLISHED TEST INSTRUMENTS (PHONOLOGICAL PATTERN TESTS)

WHO?	Children with speech disorders (generally preschool to school-age)
WHAT?	Published phonological pattern tests
WHY?	To identify the phonological error patterns in the speech of preschool to school-age children
HOW?	Administer standardized tests according to the individual test's instructions

- See Table 2–6 for a list of published phonological pattern tests that includes information regarding (1) the type of sample, (2) the sample size, and (3) the appropriate ages for test selection.

TABLE 2–6   List of Published Phonological Pattern Tests

Tests	Type of Sample	Sample Size	Appropriate Ages
Assessment of Phonological Processes-Revised (APP-R) Barbara Williams Hodson, 1986; Pro-Ed	words	107 items	3–12 years
Bankson-Bernthal Test of Phonology (BBTOP) Nicholas Bankson and John Bernthal, 1990 Riverside Publishing Co.	words	50 words	3.0–9.11 years
Khan-Lewis Phonological Analysis (KLPA) Linda Khan and Nancy Lewis, 1986; AGS	words	50 words	2–5.11 years

Tests	Type of Sample	Sample Size	Appropriate Ages
Natural Process Analysis (NPA) Lawrence Shriberg and Joan Kwiatkowski, 1980; John Wiley	spontaneous speech sample	80 words	
Phonological Assessment of Child Speech (PACS) Pamela Grunwell, 1986; College-Hill Press	spontaneous speech	100 words (min.) 200–250 words preferred	preschool–school-age
Phonological Process Analysis (PPA) Fredrick Weiner, 1979; Pro-Ed	delayed imitation words	136 criteria stimulus measures assessed by 16 phonological processes	2–5 years
Smit-Hand Articulation and Phonology Evaluation (SHAPE) Ann Smit and Linda Hand, 1996; Western Psychological Services	words	80 words used to assess 108 target speech productions with 12 common phonological processes	3–9 years

PUBLISHED TEST INSTRUMENTS (COMPUTERIZED SPEECH TESTS)

WHO?	Children with speech disorders (generally preschool to school-age)
WHAT?	Published computerized speech tests
WHY?	To assess the speech skills (sound inventory and/or phonological error patterns) of preschool to school-age children
HOW?	Administer standardized tests according to the individual test's instructions

- See Table 2–7 for a list of published computerized speech tests that includes information regarding (1) the type of sample, (2) the sample size, and (3) the appropriate ages for test selection.

TABLE 2–7   List of Published Computerized Tests

Tests	Type of Sample	Sample Size	Appropriate Ages
Computerized Assessment of Phonological Processes (CAPP) Barbara Williams Hodson, 1985; Interstate Printers and Publishers	same as APP-R		

(continues)

TABLE 2–7 *(continued)*

Tests	Type of Sample	Sample Size	Appropriate Ages
Computerized Articulation and Phonology Evaluation System (CAPES) Julie Masterson and Barbara Bernhardt, 2002; Psychological Corporation	words; connected speech	46 words (Phonemic Profile); 20–100 words (Individualized Phonological Evaluation)	2 through adult
Computerized Profiling Steven Long and Marc Fey, 1994; Psychological Corporation	words; connected speech		any age
Logical International Phonetic Programs (LIPP) K. Oller and R. Delgado, 1990; Intelligent Hearing Systems	words		
Macintosh Interactive System for Phonological Analysis (ISPA) Julie Masterson and Frank Pagan, 1992; Psychological Corporation	words		any age
Programs to Examine Phonetic and Phonologic Evaluation Records (PEPPER) Lawrence Shriberg, 1986; Lawrence Erlbaum	words		

PUBLISHED TEST INSTRUMENTS (TESTS OF NON-ENGLISH PHONOLOGY)

WHO?	Non-English-speaking children with speech disorders (generally preschool to school-age)
WHAT?	Published Tests of Non-English Phonology
WHY?	To assess the speech skills of preschool to school-age children who are non-English speakers
HOW?	Administer standardized tests according to individual test's instructions Also see Goldstein (2000)

- See Table 2–8 for a list of published tests of non-English phonology that includes information regarding (1) the type of sample, (2) the sample size, and (3) the appropriate ages for test selection.

TABLE 2–8   List of Tests of Non-English Phonology

Tests	Type of Sample	Sample Size	Appropriate Ages
Assessment of Phonological Processes-Spanish (APP-S) Barbara Williams Hodson, 1986; Los Amigos Association	words		
Austin Spanish Articulation Test (ASAT) Elizabeth Carrow, 1974; Teaching Resources	words	59 items	3–12 years
Spanish Articulation Measures-Revised (SAM) Larry Mattes, 1994; Academic Communication Associates	words		school age

NON-STANDARDIZED SPEECH TEST INSTRUMENTS

WHO?	Preschool or school-aged children with a functional speech disorder
WHAT?	Non-standardized speech test that samples all English phonemes a minimum of five times in each word position and elicits potential minimal pairs and morphophonemic alternations
WHY?	In general, to complete a more thorough analysis of the child's sound system. Specifically, to complete specific phonological analyses of the child's sound system (such as assessment of productive phonological knowledge [that is, Gierut, 1988] or independent and relational analyses [cf., Williams, 1993])
HOW?	Administer the Phonological Knowledge Protocol (PKP; Gierut, 1988) or the Systemic Phonological Protocol (SPP; Williams, 1992)

- Both the PKP Protocol (Gierut, 1988) and the SPP (Williams, 1992) provide extensive opportunities to elicit each English phoneme a minimum of five times in each word position (PKP has 196 items; SPP has 245 items).

- Both instruments also provide opportunities to assess the phonemic function of sounds in a child's language through eliciting potential minimal pairs (for example, "peach" and "beach").

- Finally, both instruments elicit specific types of data in order to identify the presence of phonological rules and thus infer the nature of the child's underlying representations. For example, items such as "pig" and "piggy" are included to determine whether a child who deletes final consonants has a rule of final consonant deletion (and therefore exhibits productive phonological knowledge of the final /g/ and the final obstruent /g/ is included in his/her underlying representation) by producing the morphophonemic alternation of [pɪ] ~ [pɪgi]. A morphophonemic alternation is the occurrence of a different pronunciation of a phoneme when it occurs in a different morphemic context. If the child does not produce a morphophonemic alternation, and therefore says [pɪ] and [pɪi], then it can be determined that the child has a phonotactic positional constraint (rather than a phonological rule) that prohibits the presence of post-vocalic obstruents. In this latter case, the child would not be attributed with knowledge of the final obstruent, and the phoneme /g/ would not occur in the child's underlying representation.

- As indicated, the PKP and the SPP are very similar. The differences include (1) the elicitation of potential morphophonemic alternations word-initially on the SPP (for example, "ship" and "reship"); (2) all items represent meaningful words on the SPP; and (3) more extensive elicitation of word-initial consonant clusters on the SPP.

- The PKP is included in Gierut (1986), *NSSLHA Journal, 14*, 83–101.

- The SPP is reprinted in Appendix C.

STIMULABILITY

WHO?	Preschool or school-aged children with a functional speech disorder
WHAT?	Stimulability testing of sounds produced in error
WHY?	(1) To determine child's ability to produce errored sounds in particular phonetic contexts and with what amount of auditory, visual, and tactile support; (2) to identify phonetic versus phonemic error types; and (3) to make clinical decisions regarding target selection (see Research Support)
HOW?	Administer formal or informal stimulability tests

- Several published sound inventory tests include stimulability testing (for example, the *Goldman-Fristoe 2* Sounds-in-Isolation subtest). This subtest assesses stimulability in different phonetic contexts (isolation, syllable, word, and sentence).

- Unpublished stimulability tests can also be used, such as Powell, Elbert, and Dinnsen's (1991) adaptation of the Carter and Buck (1958) Nonsense Syllable Task. In this task, the stimulability of individual sounds is assessed in isolation and in a series of nine different syllables that include the target in pre-, inter-, and post-vocalic syllables in three vowel contexts. For example, the stimulability of [s] would be assessed in the following 10 contexts:

Isolation: [s]   [si]   [isi]   [is]

[su]   [usu]   [us]

[sɑ]   [ɑsɑ]   [ɑs]

From this test, a stimulability score can be calculated for each sound on the basis of a percentage of correct productions across the 10 contexts in which the target was assessed.

Research Support

Powell, Elbert, and Dinnsen (1991) report that intervention on nonstimulable sounds will likely result in the child learning that sound plus other stimulable sounds. Intervention on stimulable sounds will likely result in more limited generalization to the trained sound and its cognate, however, but not to other sounds.

Miccio, Elbert, and Forrest (1999) report that nonstimulable sounds are least likely to change without treatment, whereas stimulable sounds appear to indicate that the sounds are being acquired naturally. Miccio et al., therefore, recommend that nonstimulable sounds be given priority in selecting targets for intervention.

INTELLIGIBILITY RATINGS

WHO?	Preschool and school-aged children with speech disorders
WHAT?	Intelligibility rating scales to judge how intelligible a child's speech is to unfamiliar listeners (see Research Support)
WHY?	(1) To quantify a child's speech intelligibility and (2) to document pre- and post-treatment changes in the child's speech for accountability purposes
HOW?	Administer one of the following rating scales

- Although judgments about intelligibility and severity might be correlated, they represent two different indices regarding an individual's speech. For example, a child might have a severe resonance disorder, but his/her speech is still intelligible.

- Typically, a panel of at least two and no more than five listeners listen to an audio or videotaped segment of a child's speech (either single-word or connected speech). The listeners can be familiar (clinician, teacher, or family members) or unfamiliar (other SLPs). It is important to specify who the listeners (judges) were who rated the child's speech. Obviously, familiar listeners' ratings would be higher than the ratings from unfamiliar listeners.

- Listeners are asked to rank the intelligibility of the child's speech compared to his or her chronological age peers.

- Rating scales are generally simple 3-point or 5-point judgment scales (see Bleile, 1995) that include the following:
  - Intelligible—Intelligible if the topic is known—Unintelligible (3-point scale)
  - Completely intelligible—Mostly intelligible—Somewhat intelligible —Mostly unintelligible—Completely unintelligible (5-point scale)

- The judges' scores are averaged to derive a composite intelligibility rating score.

- A comparison of 19 different intelligibility measures described by Kent, Miolo, and Bloedel (1994) is presented in Appendix D. Kent et al. described these procedures according to one of five categories that differed with regard to the emphasis of the analysis; in other words, phonetic versus phonemic and word level versus continuous speech. Although many of these procedures were developed for other populations of speakers with disordered speech (such as hearing impairment, dysarthria, or alaryngeal speech), most of the procedures can be used to evaluate the intelligibility of child speakers with speech disorders.

Research Support

Kent, Miolo, and Bloedel (1994) listed eight factors reported by Connolly (1986) that influence clinical evaluation of intelligibility. These include:

- loss of phonological contrasts

- loss of contrasts in specific environments

- extent of homonymy that results as a consequence of the loss of phonological contrasts

- amount of difference between the target sound and the speaker's realization of the target

- frequency of occurrence of the errored sound in the target language

- consistency of the errored production

- familiarity of the listener with the speaker's speech

- context in which the communication occurs

Research Support

Weston and Shriberg (1992) reported on the general contextual and linguistic variables related to speech intelligibility in children and concluded that articulation variables alone cannot account for all the breakdowns that result in communication.

SEVERITY RATING SCALES

WHO?   Preschool and school-aged children with speech disorders

WHAT?   Severity rating scales to judge the severity of the child's speech disorder

WHY?   (1) To quantify a child's speech severity; (2) to document pre- and post-treatment changes in the child's speech for accountability purposes; (3) to determine eligibility for clinical services

HOW?   Administer one of the following severity rating scales

- Similar to the intelligibility rating scales, a panel of familiar or unfamiliar listeners judge a segment of the child's recorded (audio or videotaped) speech (single word or connected speech).

- Bleile (1995) described a 4-Point Clinical Judgement Scale of Severity:

  - 4-Point Clinical Judgement Scale of Severity includes the following four points:

    No disorder—Mild disorder—Moderate disorder—Severe disorder

  - An average score of 3.5 is often required to provide clinical services.

- In addition to this perceptual scale of judged severity, there are quantitative measures of severity. Probably the most commonly used measure is Percentage of Consonants Correct (PCC), first described by Shriberg and Kwiatkowski (1982). PCC is the total number of consonants judged to be correct divided by the total number of consonants in the sample. The calculated PCC values represent an ordinal severity scale that ranges from mild to moderate. See specific values in Table 2–9.

- Shriberg (1993) described the Articulation Competence Index (ACI) as another measure for quantifying severity that is particularly well suited for children whose speech errors are primarily speech sound distortions. To obtain the ACI score, the examiner must first calculate a Relative Distortion Index (RDI), which is obtained by dividing the total number of distortion errors in a sample by the total number of articulation errors. The ACI is then calculated as PCC + RDI divided by 2.

- The Phonological Deviancy Score (PDS) derived from Hodson's *APP-R* also corresponds to a severity rating. See specific values in Table 2–9.
- Finally, a rough index of phonological severity is Edwards' (1992) Process Density Index (PDI). This metric quantifies the occurrence of multiple phonological processes that affect a single sound change. PDI represents the average number of phonological processes that are used per word. It is calculated by adding the total number of phonological processes that occurred for all words in a sample and dividing by the total number of words. The premise of this measure is that the higher the PDI, the more severe the speech disorder.

TABLE 2–9

PCC Severity Ratings (Shriberg and Kwiatkowski,1982)		APP-R PDS Severity Ratings (Hodson, 1986)	
Mild	85–100%	Mild	1–19 points
Mild-Moderate	65–84.9%	Moderate	20–39
Moderate-Severe	50–64.9%	Severe	40–59
Severe	< 50%	Profound	60+

DIALECTAL VARIATIONS

WHO?	Children who speak dialectal variations of Standard American English (SAE)
WHAT?	Dialectal variations of SAE that are associated with a particular region, social class, or ethnic group
WHY?	To provide nonbiased speech assessments in differentiating children with dialectal differences from those with speech disorders
HOW?	Determine nonstandard dialect from a speech disorder. See also Goldstein (2000)

- Presence of a nonstandard dialect (or *speech difference*) does not necessarily imply a *speech disorder*
- A speech difference refers to the speaker's first dialect (D_1) or first language (L_1).
- Speakers of a nonstandard dialect can often shift (code mix or code switch) from $D_1 – D_2$ or $L_1 – L_2$.
- A child speaking a nonstandard dialect can also present with a speech disorder.
- Proctor (1994) states that a speech disorder is determined when one of the following three conditions is present:
  - The child's intelligibility is reduced to speakers within the child's speech community.
  - The child misarticulates sounds that are similar in both SAE and D_1 or L_1.
  - The child produces idiosyncratic patterns that are not characteristic of D_1, L_1, SAE, or of the code mixing or code switching processes.

- Examples of nonstandard dialects spoken in the United States include:
  - African-American English
  - Appalachian English
  - Ozark English
  - Mexican American English
  - Caribbean English

CHARACTERISTICS OF AFRICAN-AMERICAN ENGLISH (AAE)

WHO? Child speakers of African-American English
WHAT? Phonological characteristics of AAE
WHY? To appropriately assess a speech disorder from a speech difference
HOW? Compiled from Iglesias and Goldstein (1998) and Cole and Taylor (1990).

- AAE consists of the following phonological rules relative to SAE (Table 2–10):

TABLE 2–10

AAE Phonological Rules	Examples	
Word-final cluster reduction	"test" ~ "tes"	[tɛst] ~ [tɛs]
Stopping of word-initial interdentals	"they" ~ "dey"	[ðe] ~ [de]
	"thought" ~ "taught"	[θɑt] ~ [tɑt]
Substitution of f/θ and v/ð intervocalically	"nothing" ~ "nofing"	[nʌθɪŋ] ~ [nʌfɪŋ]
	"bathing" ~ "baving"	[beðɪŋ] ~ [bevɪŋ]
Substitution of f/θ word-finally	"south" ~ "souf"	[saʊθ] ~ [saʊf]
Substitution of n/ŋ word-finally	"swing" ~ "swin"	[swɪŋ] ~ [swɪn]
Vowelization of [ɚ]	"sister" ~ "siste"	[sɪstɚ] ~ [sɪstə]
Deletion of [l] in word-final clusters	"help" ~ "hep"	[hɛlp] ~ [hɛp]
Substitution of [ɪ] for [ɛ] before nasals	"pen" ~ "pin"	[pɛn] ~ [pɪn]
Deletion of nasals word-finally with nasalization of the preceding vowel	"moon" ~ "moo"	[mun] ~ [mũ]
Devoicing of consonants word-finally	"bed" ~ "bet"	[bɛd] ~ [bɛt]

CHARACTERISTICS OF APPALACHIAN ENGLISH (AE)
AND OZARK ENGLISH (OE)

WHO? Child speakers of AE or OE
WHAT? Phonological characteristics of AE and OE
WHY? To appropriately assess a speech disorder from a speech difference
HOW? Adapted from Goldstein (2000)

- AE and OE consist of the following phonological characteristics (Table 2–11):

TABLE 2–11

Phonological Characteristics of AE / OE	Examples	
Epenthesis in word-final clusters	"ghosts" ~ "gostas"	[gosts] ~ [gostəs]
Intrusive [t]	"once" ~ "once-t"	[wʌns] ~ [wʌnst]
Stopping of interdentals	"thought" ~ "taught"	[θɑt] ~ [tɑt]
	"they" ~ "dey"	[ðe] ~ [de]
Initial deletion of [w]	"will" ~ "ill"	[wɪl] ~ [ɪl]
Deletion of initial unstressed syllables	"aloud" ~ "loud"	[əlaʊd] ~ [laʊd]
Insertion of initial [h]	"it" ~ "hit"	[ɪt] ~ [hɪt]
Deletion of [r]	"throw" ~ "thow"	[θro] ~ [θo]
	"carry" ~ "ca-y"	[kæri] ~ [kæi]
Deletion of [l] before labials	"wolf" ~ "wof"	[wʊlf] ~ [wʊf]

DEVELOPMENTAL APRAXIA OF SPEECH (DAS)

WHO? Children who appear to have difficulty with the motor aspects of speech production
WHAT? DAS, also referred to as developmental verbal apraxia (DVA), developmental verbal dyspraxia (DVD), developmental articulatory dyspraxia, or apraxia of speech in children (AOSc), but most recently referred to as child apraxia of speech (CAS)
WHY? Two reasons: (1) to understand the current controversy surrounding this diagnosis and its treatment implications for children; (2) to differentially diagnose speech disorders in children and thereby avoid misdiagnosis
HOW? See Velleman (2003)

One of the challenges in understanding speech disorders is to appropriately distinguish impairments of phonology from impairments of motor control.

- Possibly, impairments at both levels coexist in some speech disorders (Kent, 2000).
- This challenge is increased by the fact that speech is an extraordinary and unique motor skill. Speech is faster than any other discrete human motor activity, with the ability to produce up to 6–9 syllables/second. This task involves more motor fibers than any other human mechanical activity (Kent, 2000).

What Is CAS?

- Recently, Odell and Shriberg (2001) suggested the use of the term "suspected apraxia of speech in children (AOSc)" to distinguish it from the conventional, unmarked term "AOS" for adults with apraxia of speech. Childhood apraxia of speech (CAS) is the most currently used term.
- The word "apraxia" comes from the word "praxis," which means the ability to plan volitional movement.
- Therefore, apraxia means an inability to plan volitional movement.
- It was first described by two classic studies by Rosenbek and Wertz (1972) and Yoss and Darley (1974) as a speech disorder in children that supposedly shared similar features to the acquired apraxia of speech in adults.
- It is a term that has emerged primarily as a descriptive diagnosis, because a particular focal deficit in anatomical, physiological, or biochemical function has yet to be identified (Yorkston, Beukelman, Strand, and Bell, 1999).

What Are the characteristics of CAS?

- According to Davis, Jakielski, and Marquardt (1998), the following are the speech characteristics of CAS:
  - Limited consonant and vowel inventory
  - Frequent omission errors
  - High incidence of vowel errors*
  - Inconsistent articulation errors*
  - Altered suprasegmental characteristics*
  - Increased errors on longer units of speech
  - Significant difficulty imitating words and phrases
  - Predominant use of simple syllabic shapes

*These characteristics are considered to be differential diagnostic markers in assessing CAS.

What Is the Controversy Surrounding CAS?

- Lack of a diagnostic marker for CAS
- No specific set of characteristic symptoms has been identified (Yorkston et al., 1999)

- Currently, there is no single feature or combination of features that definitely confirms the diagnosis of CAS.
- According to Hall, Jordan, and Robin (1993), "The characteristics on which the diagnosis is made are not unique to CAS since they can be used to diagnose children with functional phonological disorders" (p. 337).
  - Not all children with "presumed CAS" exhibit the differentiating diagnostic characteristics.
  - The characteristics are not mutually exclusive and overlap with characteristics of a phonological impairment.
  - Early CAS children often resolve into a phonological delay.
- CAS is frequently associated with other disorders that occur with motor planning problems, such as PDD, cognitive delays, and hearing loss.
- According to Davis et al. (1998), CAS is frequently overdiagnosed. In their study, 75% of the children referred as CAS were misdiagnosed.

What Are the Implications of CAS Versus Phonological Impairment (PI)?

- It re-establishes the phonetic ~ phonemic interaction of speech disorders.
- The diagnosis (CAS ~ PI) has implications for intervention.
  - Treatment for CAS typically includes a motor-based approach, which follows a sequential pattern that progresses from simple to complex speech tasks.
  - An inherent problem with this diagnosis and treatment plan is the fact that efficacy data are rare or nonexistent (cf., Kent, 2000).
  - Other studies, such as Forrest and Morrisette (1999), have questioned CAS as a separate clinical entity by identifying the same "diagnostic markers" in children with phonological impairment. They concluded that either the feature retention patterns claimed to differentially diagnose CAS were invalid or that the children in their study who had been identified as PI were in fact CAS. If the latter were correct, then those children benefited from a linguistic-based intervention approach.
- In summary, efficacy data will provide essential information in the differential diagnosis of these children with suspected CAS. Perhaps these children fall on one end of a continuum that represents a speech disorder that involves a phonetic-phonemic impairment. Without efficacy data or other treatment options available for children with a diagnosis of CAS, we might unfortunately perpetuate Hall's (2000) claim that "we need to think of DAS as a lifelong communication problem" and that "attainment of *totally* 'normal' speech skills may be unrealistic" (p. 180).

SECTION

ANALYSIS PROCEDURES

● ●

We discuss analysis procedures separately from assessment procedures because they serve different purposes. As we discussed in the previous chapter, *assessment* identifies whether a speech disorder exists relative to a child's chronological-age peers. It determines the need for intervention and might also assess the severity of the disorder. Little information, however, is obtained regarding specific treatment goals or intervention plans. That is the objective of an *analysis* of disordered sound systems. Phonological analyses provide detailed information regarding the nature of the speech disorder, or as Grunwell (1997) claims, to identify "the order in the disorder." From a phonological analysis, clinical decisions can be made regarding appropriate target selection and intervention methods to be used.

Different analysis procedures are available to SLPs. Some are geared more toward describing mild to moderate speech disorders while others are more appropriate in analyzing severe to profound speech disorders. This chapter will provide a framework for phonological analyses, describe different analysis procedures, and conclude with a comparison of three different analyses in the description of one child's sound system.

COMPONENTS IN A PHONOLOGICAL ANALYSIS

WHO?	Speech-language pathologists who analyze children's sound systems
WHAT?	*System, Structure,* and *Stability* are the three components that comprise a phonological analysis of a child's sound system
WHY?	To provide a thorough analysis of disordered sound systems
HOW?	Determine the phonetic inventory, rules and organization, and consistency of a child's sound system

- Grunwell (1997) suggests that the primary objective of a phonological analysis is to *identify, describe,* and *classify* sound differences between a child's sound system and the target sound system.
- To accomplish this objective, Grunwell (1997) states that there are three key components of a phonological analysis: system, structure, and stability.
  - *System* includes the inventory of different sounds produced by the child. The sounds comprised in the system function contrastively to signal differences in meaning. For example, "*pat*" and "*bat*" differ in only one sound, but that difference signals a difference in meaning.
  - *Structure* refers to the rules and organization of the sound system. The structure of a sound system specifies the distribution and combination of sounds within a language. For example, the sound rules of English specify that the velar nasal [ŋ] cannot occur word-initially and that only certain consonant combinations are permissible (for example, [pl, bl, kl, gl] are permissible, but not *[tl, dl]).
  - *Stability* refers to the predictability of the speaker's systemic and structural patterns or organization of his or her sound system. The inventory of sounds (system) and the rules that govern the distribution and combination of sounds (structure) provide the organization and therefore the predictability of a "phonology."
- These three components provide a framework for any phonological analysis of children's speech.

RELATIONAL ANALYSIS

WHO?	For children (typically toddler through school-age) who have speech disorders
WHAT?	Comparative description of a child's sound errors to the adult target
WHY?	To describe and classify a child's error productions relative to the adult target
HOW?	Sound-by-sound analysis or pattern analyses

- Most phonological analyses that SLPs complete on children's speech are relational analyses.
- Relational analyses provide a description of the child's sound errors *in relation* to the adult standard.

- Relational analyses make a one-to-one comparison of the child's production to the adult target and describe the differences with regard to SODA (substitution, omission, distortion, and addition), phonological processes, distinctive features, PVM (place-voice-manner) descriptions, phonological rules, or phoneme collapses.

- Because relational analyses describe only the sounds produced in error, they are also referred to as an *error analysis* of the child's speech.

- Some common relational phonological analyses include phonological process analysis and place-voice-manner analysis.

- Generally, relational analyses are based on shorter, single-word elicited samples and/or conversational speech.

- A relational analysis, such as a phonological process analysis or a PVM analysis, can be completed from the whole-word transcriptions of a standardized sound inventory test. There are also standardized phonological process analyses, as described in Table 2-6.

- Relational analyses might be more appropriate to use with children who have mild to moderate speech disorders because their sound systems are more intact and tend to have fewer idiosyncratic or unusual phonologic rules.

INDEPENDENT ANALYSIS

WHO?	For children (typically toddler through school-age) who have speech disorders
WHAT?	Description of a child's sound system as an *independent*, self-contained sound system
WHY?	To describe what a child can do in terms of a self-contained sound system
HOW?	Determine the phonetic/phonemic inventories, syllable structure, distribution of sounds, and phonologic rules

- An independent analysis is a more recently developed type of analysis that examines a child's sound system *independently* of the adult sound system.

- The child's speech is described as a unique, independent, self-contained sound system that considers the child's sound system as the "primary language."

- An independent analysis describes what sounds the child produces regardless of accuracy relative to the adult target.

- An independent analysis includes a description of the child's (1) phonetic inventory, (2) syllable structure, and (3) distribution of sounds in his or her language.

- An independent analysis describes what the child *does* as opposed to what he or she *does not* do relative to the adult target (in other words, relational analysis).

- Usually, an independent analysis is completed in conjunction with a relational analysis.

- Some phonological analyses that incorporate an independent analysis include the Assessment of Productive Phonological Knowledge (PPK; Gierut, 1988; Williams, 1991); Systemic Phonological Analysis of Child Speech (SPACS; Williams, 2001); and non-linear phonological analyses, such as autosegmental (Goldsmith, 1976; 1990), lexical (Goldsmith, 1990), metrical (Goldsmith, 1990), feature geometry (McCarthy, 1988; Sagey, 1986), and optimality theory (Paradis, 1988; Barlow and Gierut, 1999).

- Phonological analyses that incorporate both an independent and relational analysis are generally based on longer samples of elicited words (100–250 words) and are typically used with children who exhibit moderate to severe speech disorders.

- The combination of an independent and relational analysis provides a more complete and thorough description of a child's speech.

- A fuller understanding of a child's speech is possible if we first understand the structure and organization of his or her own system (independent analysis).

- Information about the child's own sound system then provides a basis for relating the child's system to the adult system (relational analysis) in order to determine how the two sound systems (in other words, child:adult) are aligned.

PHONOLOGICAL PROCESS ANALYSIS: A RELATIONAL ANALYSIS

WHO?	For children who are at a rule-based stage of phonological acquisition (generally at least age 3) with a mild to moderate speech disorder
WHAT?	A type of relational, or "error," analysis that involves a non-standardized, phonological process analysis of a child's whole-word phonetic transcriptions
WHY?	(1) To provide a description of the error patterns that are present in a child's speech; (2) to identify potential targets for intervention
HOW?	Use standardized or nonstandardized phonological process analysis procedures

- Although there are a number of commercial phonological process tests available, research has demonstrated that an informal phonological process analysis that is independent of a closed set of processes was better in identifying children's error patterns than the published tests (see Research Support).

- Edwards (1994) suggested some guidelines for using a non-standardized phonological process analysis that included:

  - Using a representative speech sample of 50–100 words

  - Completing whole-word phonetic transcriptions

- The *Goldman-Fristoe Test of Articulation 2 (GFTA-2)* (Goldman and Fristoe, 1999) is commonly used as the basis for a non-standardized phonological process analysis.

- The non-standardized phonological process analysis described here will incorporate general procedures that are common to all such commercial tests without utilizing the procedures of any one particular test.

- A list of common phonological processes was compiled from phonological processes common to many commercial tests. This list is included in Table 3–1. As indicated in this table, phonological processes can be divided into four categories:

  1. *Deletion processes* in which a sound segment or syllable is deleted from the adult target

  2. *Substitution processes* in which one sound segment is replaced by another

3. *Assimilation processes* in which one sound segment influences the production of another sound to make it more similar to it in terms of place, voice, or manner

4. *Idiosyncratic processes* include sound changes that are unusual or atypical, such as [hɪp] for "ship."

TABLE 3–1   List of Common Phonological Processes

Structural Processes (Deletion Processes)

Process	Example
Final Consonant Deletion (FCD): Deletion of a consonant at the end of a word.	hot [hɑ]
Initial Consonant Deletion (ICD): Deletion of a consonant at the beginning of a word.	hot [ɑt]
Cluster Reduction (CR): Deletion of one or more consonants in a consonant cluster.	stop [tɑp]; squirrel [kɜʊ]
Weak Syllable Deletion (WSD): Deletion of an unstressed syllable.	telephone [tɛfon]
Consonant Deletion (CD): Deletion of an intervocalic consonant.	Santa [sæə]

Simplification Processes (Substitution Processes)

Process	Example
Stopping (ST): Substitution of a stop for an affricate or fricative.	cheese [tiz]; soap [top]
Fronting (FR): Substitution of an alveolar for a palatal or velar.	ship [sɪp]; gum [dʌm]
Backing (BA): Substitution of a velar or palatal for an alveolar.	top [kɑp]
Gliding (GL): Substitution of a glide for a liquid.	read [wid]
Vocalization (VO): Substitution of a vowel for a liquid.	scissors [sɪzʊz]; shovel [ʃʌvo]
Denasalization (DN): Substitution of an oral consonant for a nasal.	mop [dɑp]
Deaffrication (DA): Substitution of a fricative for an affricate.	peach [peʃ]
Apicalization (AP): Substitution of an apical consonant for a labial.	bee [di]
Labialization (LAB): Substitution of a labial consonant for a lingual.	thumb [fʌm]

(continues)

TABLE 3–1 *(continued)*

Simplification Processes (Substitution Processes)

Process	Example
Glottal Replacement (GR): Substitution of a glottal stop for a consonant in the middle or end of a word.	coat [koʔ]
Idiosyncratic (ID): Unusual or atypical substitution.	car [sɑr]

Assimilation Processes and Whole Word Processes

Velar Assimilation (VA): Substitution of a velar for a nonvelar when the word contains another velar.	cat [kæk]
Labial Assimilation (LA): Substitution of a labial for a nonlabial when the word contains another labial.	pot [pɑp]
Nasal Assimilation (NA): Substitution of a nasal for an oral consonant when the word contains another nasal.	mop [mɑm]
Prevocalic Voicing (PV): Substitution of a voiced sound for a voiceless, when followed by a vowel in the same syllable.	chimney [dɪmni]
Devoicing (DV): Substitution of a voiceless consonant for a voiced.	dog [dɑk]; zip [sɪp]
Reduplication (RD): Duplication of a stressed syllable within a word.	bottle [bɑbɑ]
Epenthesis (EP): Insertion of a sound in a word.	athlete [æθəlit]
Metathesis (ME): Reversal of two adjacent segments within a word.	ask [æks]
Coalescence (CO): Combination of two adjacent sounds resulting in two sounds being substituted with one.	sweep [fip]

- Important points to know before beginning a phonological process analysis include:
    1. *In general,* each phonological process changes one aspect of consonant production (place, voice, or manner).
    2. *Process ordering* is required when one sound error involves several different phonological processes. In this case, the application of multiple phonological processes in a sequential manner is required in order to account for all the

changes that are present relative to the adult target. Thus, the sequential application of processes is referred to as *process ordering*.

- An example of process ordering is shown as follows for a child's production of [dæt] for the target word "fat":

/fæt/	adult target
[pæt]	stopping
[tæt]	apicalization
[dæt]	prevocalic voicing

- Edwards (1992) described the occurrence of multiple processes affecting a single sound as *process density*. The further a child's production is removed from the adult target, the more phonological processes there are affecting that production. Edwards devised a metric to reflect the average number of processes that is used per word, called *process density index* (PDI). This rough measure of phonological severity is calculated by adding the total number of phonological processes that occurred for all words in a sample and dividing by the total number of words. The higher the PDI, the more severe the speech disorder. Caution should be exercised when using PDI as a severity measure, however, because all processes are given equal weight or value. For example, a common substitution process of stopping, such as t/s, is given the same value as an idiosyncratic substitution, such as w/s. Obviously, idiosyncratic errors will negatively impact intelligibility and thus increase the severity of the speech disorder—more so than the common substitution error.

- An exception to process ordering is the presence of unusual or idiosyncratic error productions, such as [l] for several different target sounds /w, s, ʃ/. In this instance, it is better to label all such unusual substitutions as idiosyncratic rather than try to apply numerous phonological processes to account for this unusual error pattern.

3. More than one phonological process can be used to label an error. For example, a child's production of [ʃɪp] for "sip" could be labeled as backing or palatalization. Either process would be correct; however, the process of palatalization provides a more precise description of what the child is doing rather than the broader and more vague process of backing.

- The following procedures are involved in completing a non-standardized phonological process analysis:

1. In order to examine the child's productions *in relation* to the adult target, the first step is to broadly transcribe the adult target for each test item. Note: The *GFTA-2* provides this first step on the response form.

2. Systematically list all phonological processes that occur in the child's production in a sequential fashion. Continue until all processes have been listed that account for the differences between the child and adult productions. An example might help illustrate this step:

Adult target	/fiŋgɚ/	"finger"
	piŋgɚ	stopping
	tiŋgɚ	apicalization
	diŋgɚ	prevocalic voicing
	diŋgʊ	vowelization

Notice in this example that target f ➔ d involved the application of three different phonological processes (stopping, apicalization, and voicing), which changed the manner, place, and voicing of the target. Thus, each process only changed one aspect of consonant production. In this example, the PDI would be 4; in other words, four different phonological processes operated on this one word. This situation indicates that the child's production was further removed from the target than would be indicated if the child had produced "finger" as [piŋgʊ], which would be a PDI of 2.

3. Organize and summarize the phonological processes identified in the analysis.

   a. A summary sheet (Williams, 2001) organizes the processes according to deletion, substitution, assimilation, and idiosyncratic processes. The Summary Sheet for the Non-Standardized Phonological Process Analysis is included in Appendix E.

   b. The number of occurrences of each process is summarized on the summary sheet.

   c. The relative ages at which the most common processes are suppressed according to Grunwell (1987) are included on the summary sheet.

4. Edwards (1994) suggested that additional information be provided to more specifically describe how the processes were applied in a sample of a particular child. Specifically, additional information would be provided about the following:

   a. Process limitation or application with regard to a class or classes of sounds

   b. Process limitation with regard to the position(s) in which the process is applied

   c. Frequency of process occurrence

   d. Consistency of the process application (in other words, which processes were the most consistent)

   e. Presence of process interaction

      Example: In the production of [diŋgʊ] for "finger," there was a process interaction of stopping, apicalization, and prevocalic voicing in the sound change of f ➔ d.

   f. Persisting normal processes

5. The final step in the phonological process analysis is selection of treatment targets.

   There are different perspectives about choosing the most appropriate phonological processes for intervention. One perspective is to select the most frequently occurring processes because these would have the greatest impact on intelligibility. Another option is to use a developmental perspective and select processes that have persisted beyond the age at which they should have been suppressed. A third option is a combination of the first two options and involves the selection of developmentally appropriate processes that are also frequently occurring.

- Advantages of a phonological process analysis:

  1. A description of the error patterns is provided.

  2. By identifying error patterns, more efficient intervention can be developed.

  3. The use of phonological process terms is common among SLPs and is easily understood by parents and teachers.

- Disadvantages of a phonological process analysis:
  1. The amount of time required to complete the analysis, particularly as compared to a similar analysis (PVM analysis) that takes less time
  2. The selection of treatment targets from the summary sheet is not always so obvious or easy. Frequently, the clinician must refer back to the analysis to determine the specific application of a phonological process.
  3. Only errors are described, and no information is provided about what the child can do. Thus, the phonological process analysis is also called an error analysis.

Research Support

Dunn (1982) compared a non-standardized phonological process analysis to several commercial phonological process analyses in the description of one child's error patterns. She found that the APP (Hodson, 1980) captured more of the child's error patterns than the other commercial analyses. None described as many of the child's error patterns, however, as the non-standardized phonological process analysis.

PLACE-VOICE-MANNER ANALYSIS: A RELATIONAL ANALYSIS

WHO?	Children at a rule-based stage of phonological acquisition (generally at least age 3) with a mild to moderate speech disorder
WHAT?	A type of relational, or "error," analysis that involves a description of error patterns in terms of the three broad parameters of consonant production; in other words, place, voice, and manner. The PVM analysis is completed on a child's whole-word phonetic transcriptions.
WHY?	(1) To provide a description of the error patterns that are present in a child's speech; (2) to identify potential targets for intervention
HOW?	Determine patterns in child's sound errors according to place, voice, and manner characteristics

- The PVM analysis describes a child's patterns of error productions on the basis of three broad categories of consonant production—place, voice, and manner of articulation.
- The PVM analysis was first described by Weber (1970) and later by Turton (1973), but it has also been used in the commercial tests of the *Fisher-Logemann Test of Articulation* (Fisher and Logemann, 1971) and the *Compton-Hutton Phonological Assessment* (Compton and Hutton, 1978).
- A PVM analysis can be completed on whole-word transcriptions from a sound inventory test, such as the *Goldman-Fristoe Test of Articulation-2*.
- The Place-Voice-Manner form is used to complete the analysis (see Appendix F). This form was developed by Thomas Powell at Indiana University in 1982. This form organizes the consonants according to manner (nasals, fricatives, affricates, liquids, and glides) along the top row of the form. Within each manner class, the consonants are listed according to place of production from the most anterior to the most posterior. Finally, voicing is indicated by shading of the voiced consonants.

- Below each consonant, there are three rows that correspond to the three syllable positions of prevocalic, intervocalic, and postvocalic. These syllable positions are listed on the left margin of the form beside each row. The clinician can choose to use word position rather than syllable position. In that case, the rows would represent word-initial, word-medial, and word-final positions. There are shaded boxes on the form to represent syllable positions (or word positions) in which a particular consonant cannot occur in English. Specifically, /ŋ/ cannot occur prevocalically (or word-initially), and glides [w, j, h] cannot occur post-vocalically (or word-finally).

- The bottom of the form contains boxes where target clusters can be included in the analysis. The clusters are divided into nasal clusters, [l] clusters, [r] clusters, [w] clusters, and [s] clusters. Examples of specific clusters are listed at the bottom of each cluster box.

- There are two final boxes on the bottom-right section of the PVM analysis form. One box provides space for the child's phonetic inventory, and the other box provides a space to summarize the predominant error patterns according to place, voice, and manner.

- Important points to know before completing a PVM analysis:

  1. Although the PVM analysis is an assessment of consonant production, vocalic [l], vocalic [r] – [ɝ, ɚ] and the family of diphthong [r]'s can be recorded in the columns for [l] and [r].

  2. Color coding is used in completing this analysis, which increases the visualization and identification of error patterns. Tally marks in blue or black ink can be used for correct productions, and a red pen can be used to write in the child's error productions. After the analysis is completed, a visible pattern of the child's errors can be easily identified.

- The following procedures are used for completing the PVM analysis:

  1. Proceed word by word from the whole-word transcriptions of the child's single-word sample. Within each word, proceed consonant by consonant until all of the child's consonantal responses have been recorded on the PVM form.

  2. Mark each consonant with the appropriate color pen (black = correct; red = incorrect) in the appropriate box for syllable or word position of the target consonant.

  3. Use tally marks to indicate multiple occurrences of a consonant, either correct or incorrect.

  4. List each error that might occur for a particular sound in a given position.

  5. Errors of deletion are indicated by the null sign, "Ø."

  6. Mark clusters in the appropriate boxes, continuing to use black pen for correct productions (such as, br – /) and the red pen to specify errors (such as, b/br – /).

  7. List the sounds produced by the child in the Phonetic Inventory box. You might choose to construct the child's phonetic inventory on the basis of independent or relational analyses. For the independent analysis, all sounds produced by the child are listed in the phonetic inventory regardless of their accuracy. For the relational analysis, only those sounds produced correctly are listed in the phonetic inventory.

– Stoel-Gammon (1987) and others suggest that a sound must occur at least two times in order to be included in the phonetic inventory. Sounds that occur fewer than two times can be listed in the inventory as marginal sounds. This situation can be indicated by placing the marginal sounds in parentheses.

8. In the last box, write the predominant error patterns that were noted according to errors of place, voice, and manner.

   For example:

Place	replaced velars with alveolars
Manner	replaced fricatives with stops
Voice	replaced voiced with voiceless
Other	replaced clusters with singletons

9. The final step in the PVM analysis is the selection of treatment targets. Similar to the phonological process analysis, a developmental or intelligibility perspective can be used, or a combination of both, for target selection.

- Advantages of the PVM analysis:
  1. Relatively simple and quick to complete
     a. PVM analysis provides similar results as a phonological process analysis and requires less time.
     b. The PVM analysis and summary sheet were together on one page, whereas the process analysis required several pages to complete and was separate from the summary sheet.
  2. The visual representation of patterns is the most functional advantage of the PVM analysis.
     a. Patterns are easily identified by the color coding of the errors and the organization of the PVM form.
     b. The selection of targets for intervention is enhanced by the visual display of the completed analysis.
  3. Because color coding is used to tally correct and incorrect consonant productions, the PVM form enables the clinician to see not only the errors in the child's speech, but also what the child is capable of doing correctly.
  4. The PVM form provides a useful tool for communicating analysis results to parents and other professionals.
  5. The PVM form is also useful in comparing pre- and post-intervention phonological analyses.
- Disadvantages of the PVM analysis:
  1. Does not identify assimilation errors
  2. Does not provide a description of deletion errors within the three broad parameters of place, voice, and manner, although these errors would be noted by the red null in the specified consonant rows or in the cluster boxes and could be specified as "Other" in the box for summary of predominant error patterns

INDEPENDENT + RELATIONAL ANALYSES

WHO?	Children at a rule-based stage of phonological acquisition (generally at age $3\,^1/_2$) with a moderate to severe speech disorder
WHAT?	Independent + relational phonological analyses of children's speech
WHY?	To provide a detailed description of a child's unique sound system as it relates to the adult sound system
HOW?	Determine the unique characteristics of a child's sound system and then compare that sound system to the adult sound system.

The combination of an independent and relational analysis provides a more complete description of the organization and rules of a child's sound system. Recall that an independent analysis examines a child's sound system as a unique, "exotic," self-contained sound system. A relational analysis then maps the child's unique sound system onto the ambient, or target, sound system.

Independent + relational analyses provide a *system-to-system* comparison of adult-to-child sound systems. This information is contrasted to the relational, or error, analyses described previously that involve *sound-to-sound* comparisons between the adult and child productions.

- Completing an independent analysis first provides the clinician with a basis for understanding the child's sound system and discovering the "order in the disorder."

- Different analyses utilize independent + relational analyses in the assessment of a child's sound system. One common analysis approach that has been frequently reported in the literature is the assessment of productive phonological knowledge (PPK), as described by Gierut (1986) and Gierut, Elbert, and Dinnsen (1987).

  1. This approach assesses productive phonological knowledge by using the tenets of standard generative phonology to infer the nature of a child's underlying representations, or competence, from the child's productions (in other words, performance) on an extensive list of words plus a conversational sample.

  2. We will describe this approach in greater detail in a following section.

- Another approach that incorporates independent + relational analyses is the Systemic Phonological Analysis of Child Speech (SPACS) described by Williams (2001).

  1. This approach incorporates aspects of Grunwell's (1987) work of mapping the child's system to the adult system.

  2. No inferences are made about a child's knowledge of the ambient sound system.

  3. This approach focuses on the description of the structure and organization of the child's sound system as it relates to the adult sound system.

  4. The mapping of the child-to-adult sound system is described in terms of phoneme collapses that are viewed as compensatory strategies developed by the child to communicate in the ambient language with his or her "own language" or limited sound system.

  5. We will describe this approach in greater detail in the following section.

SYSTEMIC PHONOLOGICAL ANALYSIS OF CHILD SPEECH (SPACS)

WHO?	For children who are at a rule-based stage of phonological acquisition (generally at least age 3) with a moderate to severe speech disorder
WHAT?	Systemic Phonological Analysis of Child Speech (Williams, 2001)
WHY?	(1) To provide a description of the organization and rules that are present in a child's sound system; (2) to identify potential targets for intervention
HOW?	Compare the child: adult sound systems in terms of phoneme collapses

General Information

- Child's entire sound system is examined as a unique, independent system and viewed as child's "own language"
- SPACS views child as an active and creative learner of the adult sound system
- SPACS maps the child's sound system to the adult's sound system by diagramming phoneme collapses.
- The collapse of several adult phonemic contrasts results in a one-to-many correspondence between the child:adult systems.

Procedures in completing a systemic phonological analysis include the following:

1. Obtaining an extensive sample of the child's productions by using an instrument such as the Systemic Phonological Protocol (SPP; Williams, 1992; and reprinted in Appendix C)
   a. This protocol elicits each target consonant a minimum of five times in each word position in which it can occur. It also provides opportunities to elicit minimal pairs and morphophonemic alternations in word-initial and word-final positions.
   b. Completing whole-word phonetic transcriptions of the child's responses

2. Organize the sample by consonant and by position.
3. Use the form for a Systemic Phonological Analysis of Child Speech (Appendix G) to complete the following steps.
4. Construct the child's phonetic inventory independently of the accuracy of his or her productions.
   a. Use Stoel-Gammon's (1987) criterion of two occurrences of a sound to be included in the inventory.
   b. Separate inventories can be constructed for word-initial and word-final phonetic inventories to provide additional information, or a composite inventory across all positions can be constructed.

5. List the distribution of sounds in the child's language.
   a. This information is Part II on the SPACS form.
   b. Indicate the presence, absence, or marginal occurrence for each consonant in each position by using the following notation:

(1) The presence of a sound in a given position is indicated by an "X."

(2) The absence of a sound in a given position is indicated by an open box, "☐."

(3) The marginal occurrence of a sound in a given position is indicated by a fraction that specifies how many times the sound was produced out of the total number of times the sound occurred in the sample. For example, "5/7" indicates that the child correctly produced the target sound in that position 5 times out of 7 opportunities.

c. Concomitantly with (b), specify what the child did in the event of marginal or absent productions of target sounds in target positions. Write above the box or fraction the sound produced by the child, or write "∅" if the child deleted the sound in a given position. This system will provide the basis for your mapping.

d. Identify patterns in the child's production of target clusters. To identify patterns in the child's production of target clusters, it will be important to classify clusters according to one of the following categories:

Stop clusters	Fricative Clusters	Broad Classification
stop + liquid stop + glide	fricative + liquid fricative + glide fricative + nasal	C + sonorant
	fricative + stop	C + obstruent

(1) Children develop different strategies to compensate for target cluster production just as they do to accommodate a limited phonetic inventory and distribution of English consonants.

(2) They might develop rules that correspond to specific target clusters, such as "stop + liquid" and "fricative + liquid" clusters. They also might, however, develop rules that are broader than these categories and that encompass all "consonant + sonorant" clusters, which would include all the above clusters except "fricative + stop" clusters. There are variations between these two extremes that reflect the level of differentiation in the child's acquisition of target clusters. Some children might have a rule that differentiates the first consonant of the cluster on the basis of place and manner. For example, "labial stops + consonants" are produced as [f] is an example of a rule that specifies the first consonant but not the second consonant of the cluster.

e. Map the child's system onto the adult's system by diagramming phoneme collapses.

(1) In typical speech, there is a one-to-one correspondence between a target sound and the speaker's production.

(2) In disordered speech, however, there is frequently a collapse of several adult phonemic contrasts to a single sound. This situation results in a one-to-many correspondence. An example is a child's production of [t] for several adult sounds, such as [t, k, f, s, ʃ, tʃ]. In this example, the child has collapsed six different adult sounds into one sound, [t]. This phoneme collapse can be diagrammed as follows:

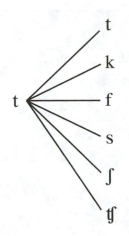

(3) To identify the phoneme collapses in a child's sound system, return to the distribution of sounds that was completed as part of (c). Part III of the SPACS form includes a section for diagramming phoneme collapses. The collapses are diagrammed by word position.

(4) In the distribution section (Part II) of the form, look for a sound that was used frequently for other target sounds in word-initial, word-medial, and word-final positions.

(5) Write the sound produced by the child in Part III under the specified position, and then diagram all the target sounds that were produced by the child with that one sound.

- Remember to list these sounds in an organized fashion; in other words, list all consonants in one manner category and by place within the manner category.

- Target clusters would be included in the collapses if the child produced the cluster with the same sound as you are diagramming the target singleton collapses.

- Continue diagramming the major phoneme collapses identified in each word position.

f. Identify organization principles that are present in the child's structure of his or her phonological system

(1) Generally, there is a correspondence between the phonetic properties of the child's production and the adult target. In the phoneme collapse diagrammed previously, the child produced a voiceless obstruent [t] for several target voiceless obstruents; that is, [t, k, f, s, ʃ, tʃ].

(2) Identification of organizational principles will lead to the identification of compensatory strategies developed by the child that correspond to the phonetic properties of the ambient sound system.

(3) Look for organized, predictable, logical, and symmetrical patterns.

g. Select targets for intervention.

(1) Williams (2000) described the guidelines for the selection of treatment targets that will have the potential for maximum reorganization and therefore have the greatest impact on intelligibility. These guidelines are discussed in detail in Chapter 4, "Guidelines for Selection of Treatment Targets: Systemic Approach."

Clinical Insight

A helpful hint in completing SPACS is organization of the analysis in terms of place and manner of consonant production.

- Organizing the child's phonetic inventory, distribution of sounds, and mapping of child:adult systems will help the clinician identify gaps in the child's inventory and patterns in their organization.
  - Organize sounds first according to manner of consonant production, such as stops, fricatives, and so on.
  - Then, organize sounds within each manner classification according to place of production, starting from the most anterior to the most posterior place of production (such as, labial, alveolar, velar for the stops).

Advantages of SPACS include the following:

- Examines correct as well as incorrect aspects of child's speech
- Provides a holistic assessment of child's sound system
- Is child-based rather than adult-based
- Describes idiosyncratic errors not captured by common phonological processes
- Phonological rules (phoneme collapses) are seen as compensatory strategies that are organized according to particular aspects of the adult sound system in terms of place, voice, and manner.
- Organizational scheme reflects unique strategies to compensate for restricted sound system

Disadvantages of a SPACS include the following:

- Although mapping of phoneme collapses is possible on smaller samples, a thorough understanding of the child's sound system requires a minimum of 100 words.
- It is time intensive to organize the sample and complete the distribution and mapping procedures. With experience, however, the analysis can generally be completed in about 30–45 minutes.

ASSESSMENT OF PRODUCTIVE PHONOLOGICAL KNOWLEDGE (PPK)

WHO?	For children who are at a rule-based stage of phonological acquisition (generally at least age 3) with a moderate to severe speech disorder
WHAT?	Assessment of Productive Phonological Knowledge (Gierut, (1986); Gierut, Elbert, and Dinnsen (1987)
WHY?	(1) To describe the nature of children's underlying representations relative to the ambient sound system in order to quantify what is known about the target language and what is unknown; (2) to identify potential targets for intervention
HOW?	Compare the child:adult sound systems in terms of productive phonological knowledge

In the mid 1980s, the assessment of productive phonological knowledge (PPK) was introduced to describe disordered sound systems. The methodology and procedures of standard generative phonology were borrowed from the field of linguistics to assess the sound systems of children with phonological disorders. As with other approaches, targets for intervention are selected on the basis of the phonological analysis. The assessment framework of PPK, however, does not select targets solely on the basis of an identified error pattern. Instead, targets are selected on the basis of the child's PPK.

Productive phonological knowledge has been defined by Elbert and Gierut (1986) as a speaker's *competence* and *performance* of the ambient sound system. Performance includes the phonetic and phonemic inventories and the distribution of the sounds in the sound system. These aspects of a sound system are contained in the surface level of representation. Evaluation of competence includes the way morphemes are stored in the speaker's mental lexicon, or underlying representation, as well as the phonological rules that operate on the underlying representations to yield the surface representation. Competence, therefore, includes the other two levels of organization: underlying representations and phonological rules.

Because underlying representations and phonological rules are abstract constructs that cannot be measured directly, they must be inferred on the basis of the child's productions. Empirical evidence is needed to infer the way in which a morpheme is stored in the underlying representations. Assessment of a child's PPK is based on production data only and does not include information about the child's speech perception abilities.

Specific types of data must be collected to determine the nature of the child's stored morphemes, or PPK. According to Elbert and Gierut (1986), three types of data must be collected: (1) elicit each target sound in each word position a minimum of five times in each position; (2) elicit potential minimal pairs; and (3) elicit potential morphophonemic alternations (in other words, variations in the way a speaker produces a phoneme when it occurs in a different context).

There are several protocols that have been developed to elicit the single word sample needed to assess PPK. One is a screening protocol developed by Maxwell and Rockman (1984) to examine a child's phonological knowledge of final consonants. A more extensive protocol is the Phonological Knowledge Protocol (PKP) developed by Gierut (1985), which contains 198 items. The Systemic Phonological Protocol (SPP; Williams, 1992) described previously is an adaptation of the PKP and includes 245 items that samples clusters as well as singletons, elicits potential morphophonemic alternations word-initially and postvocalically, and includes meaningful words.

Three components are considered when determining a child's PPK. These components include: (1) the distribution of sounds in the child's speech; (2) the presence of phonological rules; and (3) the nature of the child's underlying representations as correct (that is, adult-like) or incorrect (that is, non-adult-like).

Once the child's PPK has been assessed, it is ranked on a continuum, or hierarchy, of knowledge. According to Elbert and Gierut (1986), there are six types of phonological knowledge that can be ranked on the continuum of knowledge. These are described as follows:

Type 1: child's underlying representations are identical to the adult's underlying representations for all morphemes in all positions, and no phonological rules apply

Type 2: child's underlying representations are identical to the adult's, but phonological rules apply to change the production of the morpheme at the surface representation

Type 3: isolated incorrect production of particular fossilized forms that have been resistant to change; for example, the child produces [maezəgin] for "magazine"

Type 4: child has correct underlying representation for a target sound in some, but not all, positions in which the sound might occur; referred to as phonotactic positional constraints

Type 5: hypothesized logical possibility that has actually never yet been observed. It is a cross between Type 3 (fossilized forms) and Type 4 (positional constraints) in which a child only correctly produces a target sound post-vocalically in some "unfossilized" morphemes (Type 3) but never word-initially (Type 4).

Type 6: sounds that are represented by non-adult-like underlying representations in all positions and for all morphemes. This situation is characterized by phonotactic inventory constraints.

A summary of the knowledge types adapted from Elbert and Gierut (1985) is presented in Table 3–2.

TABLE 3–2

Knowledge Type	Underlying Representation	Target Position(s)	Target Morphemes	Rule
1	Correct	All	All	None
2	Correct	All	All	Phonological or phonetic rules
3	Correct	All	Some	Fossilized forms
4	Correct	Some	All	Phonotactic Positional Constraint
5	Correct	Some	Some	Hypothesized combination of 3 and 4
6	Incorrect	All	All	Phonotactic Inventory Constraint

Using these six types of knowledge, the child's PPK is then ranked on a continuum, or hierarchy, of knowledge. The continuum of knowledge ranges from "most knowledge" at the top to "least knowledge" at the bottom.

Dinnsen, Gierut, and Chin (1987) developed a quantitative measure that determines the proportion of a child's system that is represented by each type of knowledge ranked on the continuum. According to this procedure, one point is assigned to each target sound for each word position in which it occurs in English. Thus, a sound that occurs in three word positions (initial, medial, and final) would receive 3 points, whereas a sound that only occurs in two word positions (for example, [h]) would receive 2 points. The points are assigned to the sounds at each knowledge type along the continuum and then divided by the total number of points for all English consonants, which is 65.

Recently, Forrest, and Morrisette (1999) and Williams (2000b) have utilized this procedure to calculate the percentage of correct underlying representations (PCUR) as a measure of a child's knowledge of the ambient sound system. Knowledge types 1, 2, 3 represent adult-like, or correct, underlying representations and knowledge types 4, 5, 6 represent non-adult-like, or incorrect, underlying representations. Thus, PCUR reflects the proportion of a child's sound system characterized by knowledge types 1, 2, and 3.

Based on the assessment of a child's PPK, sounds can be selected for intervention. Several studies have demonstrated that there is a relationship between PPK and generalization learning (Dinnsen and Elbert, 1984; Elbert, Dinnsen, and Powell, 1984; Gierut, Elbert, and Dinnsen, 1986; Williams, 1991). Specifically, a child's performance will be better on phonologically "known" aspects of his or her sound system than on phonologically "unknown" aspects. Further, Gierut et al. (1986) found that training order also influenced performance. They found that children who were trained in the order of least-to-most knowledge demonstrated more system-wide changes than children who were trained in the order of most-to-least knowledge. Given the relationship between PPK and generalization learning, Gierut et al. suggested that treatment targets should be selected from those aspects of the child's system that represent the least phonological knowledge.

There are some final considerations in the assessment of a child's PPK. First, the definition and characterization of PPK are believed by some researchers to be too narrow. Tyler, Edwards, and Saxman (1990) advocate the use of perceptual and acoustic information in addition to production data in assessing PPK. Williams (1991) claimed that the definition and assessment of PPK as a dichotomous categorization of "correct" or "incorrect" cannot account for the possibility of partial knowledge that a child might have for a particular sound or class of sounds.

Secondly, it might prove more beneficial in selecting training targets to consider the child's overall phonological system rather than one aspect, such as inventory constraints or least knowledge. Consideration of the child's overall system might provide more accurate and insightful information on the nature of the child's phonological learning. The severity of the disorder might have a greater influence on phonological learning than the individual category or knowledge or the training order that is selected for treatment.

NON-LINEAR PHONOLOGY

WHO?	Speech-language pathologists; linguists
WHAT?	Non-linear phonology
WHY?	To provide a phonological description of disordered and developing sound systems that will account for prosodic effects in levels of representation that involve suprasegmental phenomena (such as stress or tone) and word-based phenomena (that is, phonotactics or the permissibility of particular consonant or vowel sequences) that are independent of the segmental representation
HOW?	Determine the organization of a child's sound system within a broader context of syllables, words, and suprasegmental phenomena

- In the 1980s, non-linear phonology was developed as an alternative to linear, or segmental, phonology in order to account for the inability of linear phonology to explain the influence of larger units above the level of the segment.

- Linear phonology's view of the sound segment as the ultimate unit for phonological rules could not account for prosodic influences, phonotactic constraints in languages, or express significant phonological generalizations that involve the larger unit of the syllable.

- Non-linear phonology's view of the syllable as a legitimate unit in phonological description is able to explain the relationships among various sizes of units that were previously restricted by linearly sequenced strings of sound segments.

- The development of non-linear phonology, therefore, represents a significant departure from the earlier linear models in that it can explain interactions that occur across various sizes of units (feature, syllable, and word) and types of units (stress, tone) in phonological representations that cannot be described by operations across a single linear sequence of phonological units.

- There are several different models of non-linear phonology, including autosegmental phonology (Goldsmith, 1976, 1990); metrical phonology (Goldsmith, 1990); lexical phonology (Goldsmith, 1990); feature geometry (McCarthy, 1988; Sagey, 1986); and optimality theory (Paradis, 1988).

- The commonality of all of these non-linear models is their emphasis on phonological *representations* rather than phonological *rules*.

- These theories are not restricted to general phonology, but they also have been recently considered with regard to their applications to phonological development and phonological disorders in children.

- In sum, non-linear phonology moves beyond descriptive accounts of children's surface patterns to an understanding of their *internal organization* and representation of their sound systems that motivates the surface patterns. If we understand the internal organization, we can better design effective interventions. It is believed that intervention is more effective by addressing and manipulating hierarchially organized *features* or *constraints*.

- Table 3–3 summarizes the comparison of linear and non-linear approaches to phonological analysis.

TABLE 3–3.   Comparison of Linear and Non-Linear Approaches to Phonological Analysis

Linear	*Non-Linear*
Segments and features are inseparable.	Segments and features are independent.
All features of a segment are equal and unstructured. • No justification for one segment to be deleted, added, or modified over another segment • No justification for a phonological rule to affect any one group of features over another • Only whole segments can be deleted or added.	Features are organized into structured bundles with minimally specified representations.
Emphasis is on formulating phonological rules.	Emphasis is on formulating phonological representations.
Unit of phonological description is the sound segment	Unit of phonological description is the syllable

CASE STUDY: COMPARISON OF THREE PHONOLOGICAL ANALYSES

WHO?	Speech-language pathologists who assess speech disorders in young children
WHAT?	A comparison of three phonological analyses of one child
WHY?	To demonstrate different assessment outcomes and compare selection of treatment targets based on each analysis
HOW?	Look at the relative benefits and drawbacks when different methods are compared

To illustrate three different phonological analyses discussed in this section, a data sample from one child, Fred, will be used. Fred is a 4-year-old boy who exhibited a severe phonological disorder. Whole-word transcriptions are provided in Table 3–4 from his single-word responses to the *Goldman-Fristoe Test of Articulation* (Goldman and Fristoe, 1986). The results from three analyses, PPA, PVM, and SPACS, will be compared with regard to their descriptions of Fred's sound system, the identification of error patterns, and the selection of treatment targets.

TABLE 3–4 Fred's Single-Word Responses on the GFTA.

Target Word	Fred's Production	Target Word	Fred's Production
house	aʊ	pencils	pɪʔkə
telephone	gɛəbo	this	ɪʔ
cup	gʌ	carrot	gʊə
gun	gʌ	orange	ɔɪwi
knife	aɪ	bathtub	bægʌ
window	wɪgo	bath	bæ
wagon	wæ	thumb	pʌm
wheel	wʊ	finger	pigʊ
chicken	gɪʔə	ring	wi
zipper	jɪpʊ	jumping	gʌʔɪ
scissors	gɪʊ	pajamas	gəwæ
duck	gʌ	plane	be
yellow	jɛo	blue	bu
vacuum	bægu	brush	bʌ
matches	mæə	drum	gʌ
lamp	æ	flag	bʷæ

(continues)

TABLE 3–4 *(continued)*

Target Word	Fred's Production	Target Word	Fred's Production
shovel	gʌʔə	Santa	dædə
car	go	Christmas tree	gəwə gwi
rabbit	wæbə	squirrel	gʊ
fishing	bɪʔɪ	sleeping	gipi
church	dʊə	bed	bɛ
feather	bɛʊ	stove	go

Phonological Process Analysis: The results of Fred's phonological process analysis are presented in Table 3–5. The results of this analysis are organized on the summary sheet in Figure 3–1. Examining the summary sheet, we can see that Fred used a number of phonological processes in his speech, including final consonant deletion (25), voicing (23), cluster reduction (17), backing (15), stopping (14), vocalization (14), and glottal replacement (7).

TABLE 3–5 Phonological Process Analysis of Fred's Single-Word Responses on the GFTA

/haʊs/	**Target**	/zɪpɚ/	**Target**
aʊs	ICD	jɪpɚ	IDIO
[aʊ]	FCD	[jɪpʊ]	VO
/tɛləfon/	**Target**	/sɪzɚz/	**Target**
dɛləfon	PV	tɪzɚz	ST
gɛləfon	BA	dɪzɚz	PV
gɛəfon	VO	gɪzɚz	BA
gɛəpon	ST	gɪɚz	CD
gɛəbon	VOI	gɪʊz	VO
[gɛəbo]	FCD	[gɪʊ]	FCD
/kʌp/	**Target**	/dʌk/	**Target**
gʌp	PV	gʌk	BA
[gʌ]	FCD	[gʌ]	FCD
/gʌn/	**Target**	/jəlo/	**Target**
[gʌ]	FCD	jɛl	WSD
/naɪf/	**Target**	[jɛo]	VO
aɪf	ICD	/vækjum/	**Target**
[aɪ]	FCD	bækjum	ST

(continues)

TABLE 3–5 *(continued)*

/wɪndo/	**Target**	bækum	CR
wɪdo	CR	bægum	VOI
[wɪgo]	BA	[bægu]	FCD
/wægən/	**Target**	/mætʃəz/	**Target**
[wæ]	WSD	mæʔəz	GR
/wil/	**Target**	[mæʔə]	FCD
[wʊ]	VO	/læmp/	**Target**
/tʃɪkən/	**Target**	æmp	ICD
tɪkən	DA	æm	CR
kɪkən	BA	[æ]	FCD
gɪkən	PV	/riŋ/	**Target**
gɪʔən	GR	wiŋ	GL
[gɪʔə]	FCD	[wi]	FCD
/ʃʌvəl/	**Target**	/dʒʌmpɪŋ/	**Target**
tʌbəl	ST (2x)	dʌmpɪŋ	DA
kʌgəl	BA (2x)	gʌmpɪŋ	BA
gʌgəl	PV	gʌpɪŋ	CR
gʌkəl	DV	gʌʔɪŋ	GR
gʌʔəl	GR	[gʌʔɪ]	FCD
[gʌʔə]	VO	/pədʒæməz/	**Target**
/kɑr/	**Target**	bədʒæməz	PV
gɑr	PV	gədʒæməz	BA
[go]	VO	gəwæmz	IDIO/WSD
/ræbɪt/	**Target**	gəwæm	CR
wæbɪt	GL	[gəwæ]	FCD
[wæbə]	FCD	/plen/	**Target**
/fɪʃɪŋ/	**Target**	pen	CR
pɪʃɪŋ	ST	ben	PV
bɪʃɪŋ	PV	[be]	FCD
bɪtɪŋ	ST	/blu/	**Target**

(continues)

TABLE 3–5 *(continued)*

bɪʔɪ	GR	[bu]	CR
[bɪʔɪ]	FCD	/brʌʃ/	**Target**
/tʃɝtʃ/	**Target**	bʌʃ	CR
tɝt	DA (2x)	[bʌ]	FCD
dɝt	PV	/drʌm/	**Target**
dʊt	VO	dʌm	CR
[dʊʔ]	GR	gʌm	BA
/fɛðɚ/	**Target**	[gʌ]	FCD
pɛðɚ	ST	/flæg/	**Target**
bɛðɚ	PV	fwæg	GL
bɛɚ	CD	pwæg	ST
[bɛʊ]	VO	bwæg	PV
/pɪntsəl/	**Target**	[bʷæ]	FCD
pɪŋksəl	BA	/sæntə/	**Target**
pɪʔkəl	GR/CR	tæntə	ST
[pɪʔkə]	VO	dæntə	PV
/ðɪs/	**Target**	dætə	CR
ɪs	ICD	[dædə]	VOI
ɪt	ST	/krɪsməs tri/	**Target**
[ɪʔ]	GR	kɪsməs tri	CR
/kɛrət/	**Target**	gɪsməs tri	PV
gɛrət	PV	gɪwəs tri	IDIO
gʊət	VO	gɪwə tri	FCD
[gʊə]	FCD	gɪwə kri	BA
/orɪndʒ/	**Target**	gɪwə gri	VOI
owɪndʒ	VO	[gəwə gwi]	GL
owɪn	CR	/skwɝl/	**Target**
[ɔɪwi]	FCD	kɝl	CR
/bæθtʌb/	**Target**	gɝl	PV
bætʌb	CD	[gʊ]	VO

(continues)

TABLE 3–5　*(continued)*

bækʌb	BA	/slɪpɪŋ/	**Target**
bægʌb	VOI	sipɪŋ	CR
[bægʌ]	FCD	tipɪŋ	ST
/bæθ/	**Target**	kipɪŋ	BA
[bæ]	FCD	gipɪŋ	PV
/θʌm/	**Target**	[gipi]	FCD
fʌm	LA	/bɛd/	**Target**
[pʌm]	ST	[bɛ]	FCD
/fɪŋgɚ/	**Target**	/stov/	**Target**
pɪŋgɚ	ST	tov	CR
pigɚ	CR	kov	BA
[pigʊ]	VO	gov	PV
		[go]	FCD

Based on this analysis, the phonological processes targeted for intervention included suppression or elimination of the processes of final consonant deletion and voicing + stopping + backing. The second target included processes that interacted together, such as voicing + stopping + backing. The specific targets to be addressed in intervention for each process include the following:

FCD　　　　　　　　　　　　　　$\emptyset \sim p / \_\_ \#$
　　　　　　　　　　　　　　　　$\emptyset \sim z / \_\_ \#$

VOI + ST + BA　　　　　　　　$g \sim \int / \# \_\_$

Place-Voice-Manner Analysis: The error patterns identified by the PVM analysis are summarized in Figure 3–2. Visual inspection of the PVM form reveals that Fred had difficulty with all three aspects of consonant production (place, voice, and manner). Fred exhibited difficulty with manner of production, specifically fricatives, affricates, and liquids. He also frequently changed place of production of target alveolars to glottals. In addition, Fred frequently produced voiced for voiceless obstruents at the beginning of words. Finally, the PVM Analysis Form also indicated that Fred frequently deleted final consonants and produced singletons for target clusters.

The targets selected for intervention based on the PVM analysis are similar to those selected on the basis of the phonological process analysis. Specifically, the targets included:

Place + Manner + Voicing　　　　　$g \sim \int / \# \_\_$
Other (final consonant deletion)　　$\emptyset \sim p / \_\_ \#$
　　　　　　　　　　　　　　　　　$\emptyset \sim z / \_\_ \#$

Non-Standardized Phonological Process Analysis Summary Sheet:

Client: _Fred_   Date: _8-15-98_

Clinician: _alw_   Age: _4-0_

	Frequency of Occurrence #times occurred # opportunities	Age of Suppression
Structural Processes (Deletion)		
Final Consonant Deletion (FCD)	28/33 = 84.8%	2:8
Initial Consonant Deletion (ICD)	4/34 = 11.8%	
Cluster Reduction (CR)	17/21 = 81%	2:8 – 3:3
Weak Syllable Deletion (WSD)	1/8 = 12.5%	3:7
Consonant Deletion (CD)	3/17 = 17.6%	
Reduplication (RD)		
Assimilation		
Labial Assimilation (LA)		
Nasal Assimilation (NA)		
Velar Assimilation (VA)		
Consonant Harmony (CH)		
Simplification Processes (Substitution)		
Stopping (ST)	9/30 = 30%	2:1 – 3:6
Fronting (FR)		
Gliding (GL)	4/8 = 50%	2:9
Vocalization (VO)	14/14 = 100%	
Deaffrication (DA)	2/7 = 28.6%	
Apicalization (AP)		

(continued)

Figure 3–1   Non-Standardized Phonological Process Analysis Summary Sheet

Summary Sheet: *(continued)*

	Frequency of Occurrence #times occurred # opportunities	Age of Suppression

Simplification Processes (Substitution) continued

Labalization (LA)		
Denasalization (DN)		
Glottal Replacement (GR)	7	
Palatalization (PL)		
Voicing (Voi)	$22/35 = 62.8\%$	2:4
Devoicing (DV)	$2/25 = 8\%$	2:4

Other Process

Idiosyncratic Processes (IP)	3
Other (Backing)	15

Summary

Classes of sounds/positions affected by processes:

fricatives (all positions)
affricates (all positions)
liquids (all positions)
stops (all positions)
nasals (all positions)

Consistency of Processes:

FCD VO
CR VOI

Process interactions:

ST + BA

Persisting Normal Processes:

FCD, CR, ST, VOI

Idiosyncratic Processes:

inconsistent (1x only): j/2, w/d3, w/m

Figure 3–1   *(continued)*

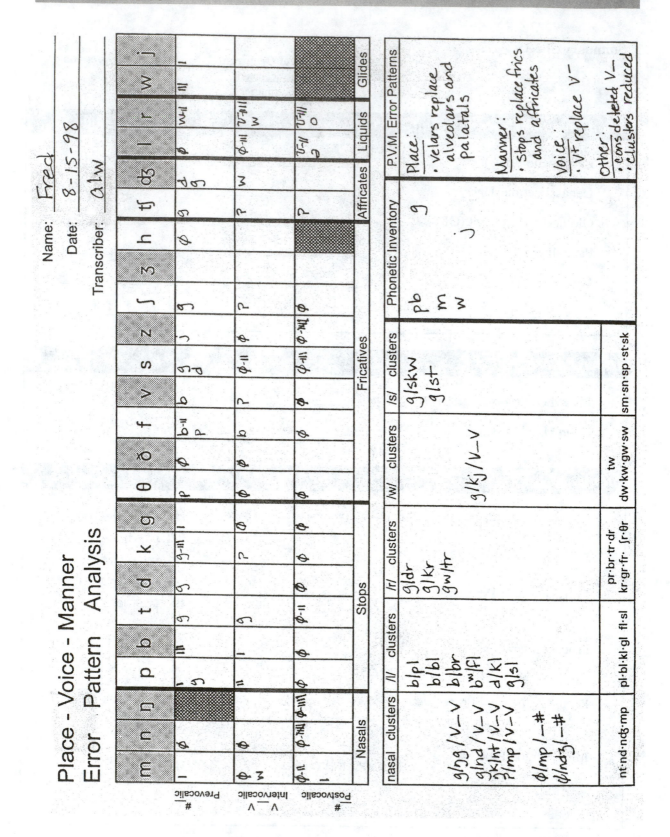

Figure 3–2   Place-Voice-Manner Error Pattern Analysis

Systemic Phonological Analysis of Child Speech: The results from the SPACS are presented in Figure 3–3. You'll notice that Fred's phonetic inventory was restricted to an incomplete set of stops, nasals, and glides. To accommodate this limited sound inventory, Fred had to collapse several adult targets into a single sound, which resulted in extensive phoneme collapses.

Systemic Phonological Analysis of Child Speech (SPACS)

Client: _Fred_   Date: _8-15-98_

Clinician: _alw_   Age: _40_

Phonetic Inventory (Systemic)	Word-Initial	Word-Final
Stops	p b g ʔ	ʔ-
Nasals	m	m
Fricatives		
Affricates		
Glides	w j	
Liquids		

Distribution of Sounds (Structural)

Stops		#___	V__V	___#	Affricates		#___	V__V	___#
	p	½ᵇ	X	□ᵠ	Affricates	tʃ	□ᵈ	□ʔ	□ʔ
	b	X	X	□ᵠ		dʒ	□ᵍ	□ᵍ	□ᵠ
	t	□ᵍ	□ᵍ	□ᵠ	Nasals	m	X	NT	X □ᵠ
	d	□ᵍ	NT	□ᵠ		n	□ᵠ	□ɔ	□ᵠ
	k	□ˢ	□ʔ	□ᵠ		ŋ		□ᵍ	□ᵠ
	g	X	□ᵠ	□ᵠ	Glides	w	X	NT	
Fricatives	f	□ᵠᵖ	□ᵇ	□ᵠ		j	X	NT	
	v	□ᵇ	□ʔ	□ᵠ		h	□ᵠ	NT	
	θ	□ᵖ	□ᵠ	□ᵠ	Liquids	l	□ᵠ	□ᵠ	□ᵛᵒʷᵉˡ
	ð	□ᵠ	□ᵠ	NT		r	□ʷ	□ᵠ	□ᵛᵒʷᵉˡ
	s	□ᵍʼᵈ	□ᵏ	□ᵠ					
	z	□ʲ	□ᵠ	□ᵠ					
	ʃ	□ᵍ	□ʔ	□ᵠ					

Clusters:

$$C + C \rightarrow C_{[g \text{ or } b]}$$

(continues)

Figure 3–3 Systemic Phonological Analysis of Child Speech (SPACS)

Mapping Child-to-Adult Systems (Phoneme Collapses)

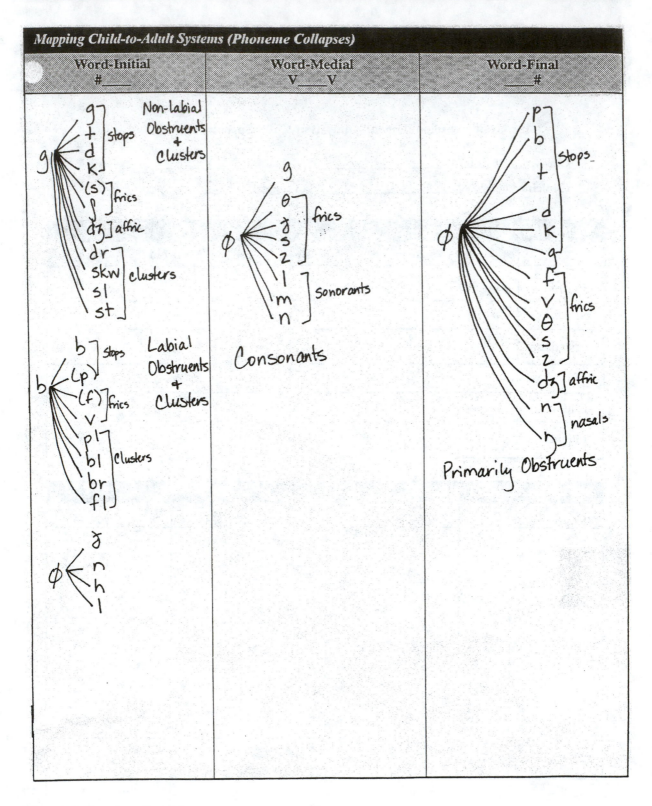

Figure 3–3 *(continued)*

Two primary phoneme collapses were identified word-initially and are shown in the diagram that follows:

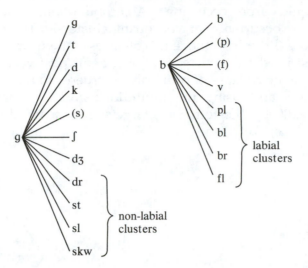

Interestingly, these collapses are mirror images of each other in terms of place (labial versus non-labial) and, roughly, manner (obstruents). Fred collapsed non-labial obstruents and clusters to /g/, and labial obstruents and clusters were collapsed to /b/. Notice the symmetry of his collapse (non-labial obstruents versus labial obstruents) and the correspondence of Fred's rule to the adult rule. Specifically, Fred produced a non-labial obstruent, [g], for target non-labial obstruents. He produced a labial obstruent, [b], for labial obstruents. These collapses suggest that Fred has organized his limited sound system according to the broad distinctions of place (labial versus non-labial) and manner (obstruents). Voicing distinctions were not consistently maintained in his sound system.

Word-finally, Fred deleted primarily obstruents, as shown in the diagram that follows.

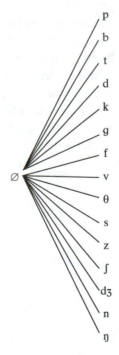

These extensive phoneme collapses reflect the phonotactic constraints that were operating on Fred's sound system. Specifically, phonotactic inventory constraints restricted fricatives, affricates, and liquids from occurring. A second phonotactic constraint, sequence constraints, restricted the occurrence of consonant clusters. These two constraints are reflected in the first two word-initial phoneme collapses. The third phonotactic constraint, positional constraint, restricted the occurrence of obstruents post-vocalically. This constraint resulted in the third phoneme collapse of primarily obstruents to null word-finally.

Based on the SPACS and using the multidimensional distance metric guidelines described by Williams (2000b), the following targets from a word-initial and word-final phoneme collapse would be likely candidates for intervention using a multiple opposition approach:

From the word-initial collapse to [g], you'll notice that a target from each obstruent class (stop, fricative, and affricate) was selected as well as a cluster from the group of clusters that were collapsed. Further, place of production was fully represented in the target selection (alveolar, palatal, and velar cluster). Similarly, for the collapse of obstruents to null word-finally, targets from each obstruent class were selected across three different places of production.

Comparison of Analyses: The two relational analyses (PPA and PVM) provided similar results despite differences in terminology. Both analyses identified errors with place, voice, and manner of production and identified deletion of final consonants and reduction of clusters to singletons. Although both analyses identified the same targets for intervention, the selection of treatment targets was much easier from the visual display of the PVM analysis than the longer summary sheets used for the phonological process analysis.

The independent + relational analysis of the SPACS, however, provided a much richer description of Fred's sound system than either of the relational analyses. From the SPACS, we also have a better understanding of Fred's phonological disability in terms of the organizational principles that he developed to compensate for a restricted sound system. Selection of treatment targets from the phoneme collapses was also easy to identify.

A comparison of the treatment targets selected from each of the analyses is summarized in Table 3–6.

TABLE 3–6 Comparison of Target Selection across Three Phonological Analyses.

PPA	PVM	SPACS
VOI+ST+BA: g ~ ʃ /#___	P+V+M: g ~ ʃ / # ___	Collapse of non-labial obstruents to [g]:

PPA	PVM	SPACS
FCD: Ø ~ p / __# Ø ~ z / __#	Other: Ø ~ p / ___ # (deletion Ø ~ z / ___ # of final consonants)	Collapse of obstruents to null:

Across the three analyses, only Ø ~ p and Ø ~ z / ___ # were the same targets selected. Although each analysis selected the error production of [g], the SPACS selected different target sounds to contrast with /g/ than the other two relational analyses.

SECTION

INTERVENTION PRINCIPLES, METHODS, AND MODELS

• •

This section includes procedures for providing intervention to children with speech disorders. The format will be the same as that in previous sections.

GOALS OF PHONOLOGICAL INTERVENTION

WHO?	Children with speech disorders
WHAT?	Goals of phonological intervention
WHY?	To establish a general foundation of phonological intervention in order to make the process of intervention planning more explicit and congruent with the established theoretical assumptions
HOW?	Facilitate cognitive reorganization of a child's sound system

The following goals of phonological intervention are adapted from Grunwell (1997):

- A child must develop a system of sound contrasts that function to signal meaningful contrasts in the target language.
- To develop these meaningful contrasts, the child must reorganize his or her sound system.
- This cognitive reorganization is based on perceived patterns of similarities and differences in order for the child to group sounds into classes and sequences into structures in the development of new rules and hypotheses.
- Therefore, the goal of intervention is to facilitate the cognitive reorganization of the child's sound system.

PRINCIPLES OF PHONOLOGICAL INTERVENTION

WHO?	Children with speech disorders
WHAT?	Principles of phonological intervention that guide the process of intervention planning
WHY?	To establish the *modus operandi* of phonological intervention
HOW?	Adapted from Grunwell (1997)

- The following principles of phonological intervention were adapted from Grunwell (1997) and include the following:
  1. Intervention is based on the phonological assessment, and the goals are defined by the phonological analysis.
  2. Intervention is based on the principle that there is "order in the disorder."
  3. The principle function of intervention is phonological reorganization.
  4. Intervention addresses the function and use of contrastive sounds as in the target language; thus, the purpose of phonological reorganization is communicative.
- Phonological reorganization is facilitated by the following:
  1. Confrontation of the child's system with the adult system through the use of contrastive word pairs
  2. Communication-centered, meaningful intervention activities
  3. Focused practice to stabilize new contrasts

GENERAL CONSIDERATIONS IN PHONOLOGICAL INTERVENTION

WHO?	SLPs who provide intervention services to children with speech disorders
WHAT?	General intervention considerations for providing intervention to children with speech disorders
WHY?	To provide appropriate intervention services
HOW?	Utilizing meaningful, focused activities that involve active participation

- Choose an intervention approach appropriate to the child's speech disability and diagnosis.
- Make intervention meaningful (rules, sounds, and stimuli).
- Be encouraging to the child's attempts and successes.
- Encourage a risk-taking atmosphere.
- Maintain an active pace that will elicit a high response rate (generally 80–100 responses in a 20–30 minute session).
- Provide immediate linguistic feedback.
- Utilize phonetic shaping and cues (auditory, visual, and tactile) as needed.
- Maximize the child's attention and focus to the new phonologic learning.
- Reduce or minimize distracting factors (for example, playing board games) during the early phases of intervention.
- Seat facing the child and decrease the distance between you and the child by having the child sit in an adult chair and you sit in the child chair.
- Maximize the therapeutic potential of antecedent and consequent events by:
  - Exaggerating the target sound in your models
  - Supplementing verbal models with physical prompts (for example, moving the treatment card out to side as you exaggerate the "long sound" [s] in the word "ssssee")
  - In the early phases of intervention, shadow the child's productions and incorporate physical prompts during his or her response in order to "set up" the child for the best possible response.
  - Providing immediate feedback contingent on the child's production (be specific, concise, therapeutic, and encouraging)
- Program for generalization by systematically reducing these supports in your models and setups, as well as to systematically introduce distracting factors, such as fading stimulus support (Costello, 1977)

TYPES OF CLINICALLY INDUCED PHONOLOGICAL CHANGE

WHO?	Children with speech disorders
WHAT?	Types of phonological change that can be induced by phonological intervention
WHY?	To understand the nature of change that occurs as a result of intervention
HOW?	Adapted from Grunwell (1997)

- There are four basic types of change that occur as a result of intervention (adapted from Grunwell, 1997). These types of induced clinical change often follow a sequence, as follows:

1. Destabilization—disruption of the original error patterns
   - Frequently results in overgeneralization of the new sound contrast to the comparison sound

- For example, a child learns [s] in [t ~ s] contrasts and begins to produce [s] for target /t/ words.

2. Innovation—introduction of a new system of sound contrasts
   - Child learns appropriate use of new sound contrast

3. Stabilization—new contrasts resolve into a stable pattern of production
   - Productions reveal a new sound contrast that is automatic rather than reflective of an articulatory routine.

4. Generalization—transfer of new phonologic learning to related pattern or phoneme collapse
   - New sound contrast is integrated into the child's phonological system as a new rule
   - Often realized as "across the board changes" to other positions and to other sounds affected by the original rule

TREATMENT CONSIDERATIONS

WHO? Children with speech disorders

WHAT? Considerations for designing phonological intervention

WHY? To consider different variables in designing appropriate phonological intervention

HOW? Select appropriate goal attack strategies, a treatment model, a treatment paradigm, and treatment materials

The following variables need to be considered in designing appropriate phonological intervention:

- Goal attack strategies: Fey (1986) described three different approaches for determining how goals will be addressed in each treatment session.
  1. Vertical Approach—one goal is taught at a time in each session until a predetermined criterion is obtained.
  2. Horizontal Approach—more than one goal is addressed in each treatment session. Multiple goals are either addressed individually or interactively.
  3. Cyclical Approach—a number of goals are addressed in a cyclical fashion, with only one goal incorporated at a time within a session.

- Number of contrasts to be trained: Williams (2000) described different contrastive phonological approaches that use either single oppositional contrasts or multiple oppositional contrasts. Single versus multiple contrasts reflects different models of phonological intervention that are discussed in more detail under "Linguistic Models of Intervention." In general, models that involve single contrasts include the following:
  1. Minimal pair therapy (cf., Weiner, 1982)
  2. Maximal oppositions (Gierut, 1989)
  3. Treatment of the empty set (Gierut, 1992)

One model of intervention incorporates multiple contrasts: multiple oppositions (Williams, 2000a; 2000b).

- Treatment paradigm: Clinicians must determine the structure of their intervention process. Included in their paradigm is the decision of whether to initiate intervention at an imitative or spontaneous level, criterion levels to determine when to proceed to more complex levels of interventions and when to terminate intervention. Williams (2000b), as well as under the section "Treatment Paradigm," describes a treatment paradigm that includes information about phases and criterion levels for a child's matriculation through intervention to dismissal.

- Treatment materials: Selection of appropriate intervention materials is a central piece of phonological intervention.

  1. There are several commercial intervention materials available. Most of these, such as *Contrasts: The Use of Minimal Pairs in Articulation Training* (Elbert, Rockman, and Saltman, 1980); *Contrast Pairs for Phonological Training* (Palin, 1992); or *Remediation of Common Phonological Processes* (Monahan Broudy, 1993), rely on the theoretical framework of phonological processes.

  2. There are software programs available for articulation and/or phonological intervention. These include *PictureGallery: Articulation and Phonology, SAILS* (Speech Assessment and Interactive Learning System), and *LocuTour: Phonology CD* and *LocuTour: Articulation CD.* It should be noted that these software programs provide limited production activities for contrasts. Either they include individual pictured representations of words for production practice, or they focus primarily on receptive activities of discrimination and identification of minimal contrasts. A software program (*Sound Contrasts in Phonology;* SCIP; Williams, 2002) is currently under development that will provide production activities of single or multiple contrastive word pairs.

  3. The third option is the traditional method of selecting or creating pictured stimuli from different resources and cutting and pasting. This method is neither time efficient or cost effective.

SELECTION OF TARGETS FOR INTERVENTION

WHO?	Children with speech disorders
WHAT?	Three different perspectives on the selection of targets for phonological intervention
WHY?	To provide different guidelines of treatment targets that will lead to the greatest amount of change in the least amount of time
HOW?	Different target selection criteria suggested by Gierut, Morrisette, Hughes, and Rowland (1996), Rvachew and Nowak (2001), and Williams (2000b)

- Williams (2000b) discussed different approaches to the selection of treatment targets for phonological intervention. These approaches are discussed in three categories:

  1. Phonetic approach
  2. Phonemic approach
  3. Functional, or systemic, approach.

Phonetic Approach to Target Selection

- The phonetic approach to target selection incorporates one or more phonetic factors in identifying potential sounds for intervention. Two of the most common phonetic factors that are considered include:
  1. developmental norms
  2. stimulability
- Both of these factors are based on the peripheral aspects of sound production with particular emphasis on relative ease of production. Both factors assume a motoric basis for sound acquisition, with easier sounds being those that are stimulable and acquired early. As a consequence, traditional approaches to target selection have used these factors in selecting sounds for remediation.

Developmental Norms

- Typically, targets selected on the basis of developmental norms assume that there is a developmental sequence of sound acquisition in which sounds are learned in a particular order. The assumption underlying the sequence of acquisition is that earlier-developing sounds are easier to learn while later-developing sounds are more difficult to acquire. It is further assumed that the acquisition of earlier-developing sounds is a prerequisite to the acquisition of later-developing sounds.
- Although the validity of these assumptions has been questioned in a study by Gierut, Morrisette, Hughes, and Rowland (1996), a more recent study by Rvachew and Nowak (2001) provided support for the traditional use of developmental norms in selecting treatment targets. Refer to Research Support in this section.
- Another concern regarding the use of developmental norms is the differences in ages of acquisition reported by various studies that result from relative small differences in methodology (see "Developmental Norms" in Section 1 entitled "Core Knowledge").
- A further concern about developmental norms is the normal variation observed in typically developing children. Studies of small groups of typically developing children have reported individual differences across children that may make it impossible to establish meaningful age norms for sound acquisition.

Research Support

Gierut, Morrisette, Hughes, and Rowland (1996) compared treatment outcomes in two groups of children in which early and later-developing sounds were selected for intervention. Their results indicated that intervention on later-developing sounds led to system-wide changes in untreated sound classes, whereas intervention on early developing sounds did not result in system-wide changes.

Rvachew and Nowak (2001) challenged these findings in a study that compared the treatment of two groups of children with moderate to severe phonological impairments. One group received intervention on early acquired sounds that were characterized as most phonological knowledge while the second group received training on later-acquired sounds that were associated with least phonological knowledge. Their results indicated that children who received treatment on early developing sounds associated with greater knowledge made significantly greater progress in intervention than children who received treatment on later-developing sounds that were characterized by little or no phonological knowledge.

Stimulability

- Another common method for target selection is on the basis of sound stimulability. Typically, it has been suggested that stimulable sounds be selected over nonstimulable sounds.

- It was believed that stimulable sounds, similar to early developing sounds, represented an easier sound for the child to learn. Conversely, nonstimulable sounds would be more difficult for the child to learn.

- This long-standing recommendation has been recently challenged by Powell, Elbert, and Dinnsen (1991) and Miccio, Elbert, and Forrest (1999). Refer to the research support under "Stimulability." Specifically, Powell et al. (1991) found that greater change occurred on nonstimulable sounds, whereas limited generalization occurred on stimulable sounds. Miccio et al. (1999) extended these findings to the predictability of change. They reported that stimulable sounds are likely to change on their own without direct intervention, whereas nonstimulable sounds are least likely to change.

Phonemic Approach to Target Selection

- More recently, a phonemic approach has been advocated for the selection of targets for phonologic intervention.

- Gierut, Morrisette, Hughes, and Rowland (1996) described phonemic factors as superordinate properties of a sound system. They suggested that greater phonologic change might result from the incorporation of higher order, or superordinate, properties. Gierut et al. discussed four phonemic factors that can be considered in selecting treatment targets. These include: (1) markedness; (2) productive phonological knowledge; (3) relation of contrastive pairs to the child's existing grammar; and (4) the phonemic complexity of contrastive pairs. Each of these factors will be discussed separately.

Markedness

- Markedness is a linguistic construct that deals with implicational relationships of phonologic properties that govern all human languages.

- A marked property of a language refers to the presence of a particular feature of a given language in which another feature is necessarily implied by the occurrence of the marked feature.

  - For example, there are languages that have both voiced and voiceless sounds, and there are languages that only have voiced sounds.

  - There are, however, no languages that only have voiceless sounds.

  - Therefore, voicing is a marked property of language in which the presence of voiceless sounds necessarily implies the presence of voiced sounds in a given language.

- Based on the markedness construct, it has been recommended that treatment should target marked properties in order to facilitate the acquisition of unmarked aspects.

  - Refer to the following Research Support for evidence of marked aspects of a sound system facilitating the acquisition of unmarked properties.

Research Support

Several studies have demonstrated that treating the marked aspects of a sound system results in the acquisition of the unmarked properties, but not vice-versa. For example, McReynolds and Jetzke (1986) found that treating voiced obstruents facilitated the acquisition of voiceless obstruents. Similarly, Dinnsen and Elbert (1984) treated the marked class of fricatives, which facilitated the acquisition of the unmarked class of stops. In another study, Elbert, Dinnsen, and Powell (1984) treated marked fricative + liquid clusters and the children acquired the unmarked stop + liquid clusters.

Productive Phonological Knowledge

- Productive phonological knowledge (PPK) refers to a speaker's underlying competence, or knowledge, of the ambient sound system.
- PPK reflects the nature of a child's stored morphemes in his or her mental lexicon based on specific types of production evidence.
- Sounds in morphemes that are stored as in the adult sound system are credited as having phonological knowledge of those particular sounds.
- Three types of evidence are required to infer that the morphemes are stored in an identical fashion to the adult underlying representations. These include:
  (1) Phonemes that are represented in all positions and in all morphemes, just as in the adult system (that is, always correct)
  (2) Phonemes that are represented in some, but not all, positions in an adult-like manner resulting from either a phonological rule that changes the correct underlying representation to a surface representation that is different from the adult form or from a phonotactic positional constraint
  (3) Phonemes that are represented in all positions in an adult-like manner in most, but not all morphemes (in other words, occasional errors)
- A study by Gierut, Elbert, and Dinnsen (1987) reported that greater system-wide change occurred when intervention was provided on "unknown" aspects of a child's phonological system than when "known" aspects were trained. Refer to the following support section.

Research Support

Additional studies have qualified the role of PPK in phonologic learning. Specifically, Dinnsen, Gierut, and Chin (1987) specified the role of PPK in a child's overall system and its impact on learning. They reported that training "least knowledge" or unknown aspects resulted in system-wide change in children who had less than 50% of their sound systems characterized as inventory constraints.

In another study by Williams (1991), the dichotomy of "known ~ unknown" was questioned with regard to the presence of partial knowledge. In that study, nine children were trained on inventory constraints, [s, r], in the context of clusters. Although all children exhibited the same level of phonological knowledge for these clusters, different learning patterns were obtained following intervention. Children who had a knowledge of producing two sequential consonants such as, [tw] for [tr], made greater gains than children who reduced target clusters to a singleton, such as, [t], or even to a third consonant, such as [f].

Relationship of Contrasting Pairs to Child's Existing Grammar

- Typically, a target is selected for intervention and contrasted with the child's error substitution.

- For example, target /s/ might be selected for intervention and contrasted with the child's error production of [t]. The contrasting pair in this example relates directly to the child's existing grammar.

- Recently, Gierut (1989; 1990) has questioned this relationship in focusing the child's attention to the need to eliminate the homonymy in his or her language. Rather, Gierut's studies have shown that homonymy is more readily eliminated when the target sound is not contrasted to the child's error substitution in a one-to-one correspondence to his or her existing grammar.

- She proposed two different approaches that select comparison sounds that are independent of the child's error substitution.

  - One approach contrasts the child's error with an independent sound that is maximally different from the target sound and is produced correctly by the child (maximal oppositions).

    - In this example, target /s/ can be contrasted with a sound that is unrelated to the child's error substitution of [t] but is produced correctly by the child. Gierut (1989) contrasted [s] ~ [w] for one child.

  - The second approach contrasts two unknown sounds with each other that are maximally different (treatment of the empty set).

    - In this approach, target /s/ would be contrasted with another errored sound that is maximally different, such as /dʒ/.

- With regard to this phonemic factor, the primary focus is on the selection of the *comparison sound* to be used in the contrastive treatment pairs and how it differs from the *target sound* in terms of distinctiveness and independence.

Phonemic Complexity

- This factor corresponds to the previous discussion of the selection of comparison sounds that are maximally distinct from the target sound.

- In studies by Gierut (1990; 1992), she demonstrated that greater phonological change occurred when the contrastive difference between the two sounds involved major class distinctions (that is, [sonorant], [consonantal], and [syllabic]) and maximal distinctive feature differences.

- Again, the focus is primarily on the nature of the comparison sound rather than on the target sound, except of course in the treatment approach of the empty set in which both sounds are target sounds.

- In summary, Gierut et al. (1996) believed that the phonemic factors, or superordinate properties, drive the subordinate, or phonetic, properties of a sound system. Therefore, the treatment of superordinate properties will facilitate the acquisition of the lower, subordinate properties of a sound system.

Functional (Systemic) Approach

- Williams (2000b) described an approach to target selection that is based on the *function* of the sound in the child's own system and its potential for having the greatest impact on phonological restructuring.

- It is not the *nature* of the sound itself, either phonetically or phonemically, that is the basis of selection.
- Rather, it is the *function* of the sound in the organization of the child's sound system.
- As noted previously, two characteristics of a phonological disorder are the multiple collapse of adult phonological contrasts in the child's system and the relationship between the phonetic properties of the adult target and the phonetic properties of the child's realization.
- Given these two characteristics, it can be seen that the collapse of sound(s) in the child's system will serve a compensatory function to organize the child's system relative to the adult system within the constraints of the child's limited sound system.
- Williams (2000a) presented two hypothetical cases in which both children collapsed several adult targets to [t] word-initially.
  - One child collapsed target voiceless obstruents (/k, tʃ, f, s, ʃ/) to [t], whereas the other child collapsed target voiceless velar stop and clusters (/k, tr, st, sk, kr, kl, kw/) to [t].
  - Notice the phonetic resemblance of the child to adult systems in each example. The child in both cases did not have the phonetic repertoire to produce all the adult targets yet produced a sound from his or her limited repertoire that was phonetically related to the adult targets.
  - Additionally, this example further shows that each child has different learning needs based on their own unique phonological organization.
- A systemic approach would examine the learning needs in each example and select targets on the basis of their function within that collapse.
  - For the first child, target selection can include [t] ~ [k, tʃ, f] to facilitate the child's learning of voiceless obstruents across a spectrum of sounds affected by the child's rule.
  - For the second child, the targets might include [t] ~ [k, tr, st] to facilitate the child's learning of velars and sequential consonant production.
- Therefore, sounds that have the potential for the greatest impact on phonological reorganization are based on a multidimensional distance metric relative to the child's phonological organization.
  - This distance metric examines the relationship of a target sound within the organization of the sound system and then selects the sound(s) for intervention, which will highlight the saliency of the new contrast(s) to be learned.
  - The distance metric identifies targets for intervention from the extremes of the child's phonologic organization along two parameters or dimensions: maximal distinction and maximal classification.
    - Maximal distinction involves the selection of a target that is the most distinct from the child's error.
    - Maximal classification is the selection of target(s) from different sound classes that are collapsed in the child's system.
- The systemic approach to target selection differs from both phonetic and phonemic approaches, which focus on the nature of the sound itself for selecting targets for intervention.
- Gierut (1990b) claimed that it is the nature of the opposition (minimal, maximal, or empty set) that is essential in shaping the course of phonological learning.

- Conversely, it is the level of the system that is considered important in inducing the greatest phonological change in the systemic approach.
- Although yet to be experimentally verified, the systemic approach to target selection might be a variable in inducing phonological change.
  - Williams (2000b) reported treatment results on 10 children in a study that examined the impact of several variables on phonological learning. One variable that potentially impacted the course of learning was the selection of treatment targets on the basis of systemic factors.

TREATMENT PARADIGM

WHO?   Children with speech disorders

WHAT? Paradigm for phonological intervention

WHY?   To provide a structured framework for making intervention decisions regarding linguistic complexity, treatment criterion levels, generalization criterion levels, and discontinuation of a goal

HOW?   Williams (2000b) described a treatment paradigm for phonological intervention

- Once a child's system has been analyzed and treatment targets have been selected, clinicians need to incorporate a paradigm within which they will implement their chosen intervention approach.
- The paradigm will provide a framework for determining criterion levels for treatment to move to more complex linguistic levels of intervention, generalization criterion levels, and when to discontinue treatment for a particular goal.
- Williams (2000b) described a treatment paradigm that can be used with word-based contrastive intervention approaches.
  - Therefore, this paradigm is flexible and can be used with minimal pair therapy (Weiner, 1981), multiple oppositions (Williams, 2000a; 2000b), maximal oppositions (Gierut, 1989; 1990), or treatment of the empty set (Gierut, 1992). Each of these approaches is described in later sections.
- The rationale underlying this treatment paradigm was described by Williams (1992) to include similar psycholinguistic principles outlined by Johnston (1984) in her FAAcTual approach for language intervention.
  - The acronym for FAAcTual represents intervention that is **F**unctional or meaningful and communicative, provides linguistic input that is **A**ppropriate to the child's developmental level and interests, allows for **Ac**tive rule discovery, and provides input that is **T**herapeutic.
  - Incorporated in the phonological intervention paradigm, these principles are included in the following:
    - Provide opportunities for the child to discover the rule that is being trained.
    - Have unusually focused therapeutic input, which reduces the child's search for the new contrast and thereby reduces demands on attention and memory.
    - Have a high proportional frequency of occurrence of the target contrast(s) in salient contexts using stress and intonation paired with physical prompts of the

new contrast to be learned (for example, contrasting long and short arm movements coinciding with the production of fricative and stop sounds).

- Incorporate the new contrast in both focused and play intervention activities in order to expose the child to the range and application of the new rule.

- Provide opportunities for the child to use the new contrast(s) in meaningful, naturalistic play activities.

- Provide the child with linguistic/communicative feedback with regard to the semantic meaning of the child's production.

- In addition to these psycholinguistic principles, an additional principle is incorporated that addresses the dual nature of phonologic learning, such as learning of the new linguistic rule (conceptual) *and* learning of the new articulatory pattern (motoric).

  - Provide focused practice on the new contrast(s) to be learned in order for the form to become automatic.

  - Generally, five contrastive sets are used in intervention with a recommended response rate of around 60–100 responses per session. Refer to the Research Support section regarding the number of treatment stimuli to be used in intervention.

- These principles were incorporated within a treatment paradigm that was designed to combine focused practice within a communicative context utilizing naturalistic play activities. A diagram of the treatment paradigm is illustrated in Figure 4–1.

- The first phases of this paradigm rely more heavily on focused practice with the initiation of intervention at an imitative level (Phase 1).

- The later phases utilize more naturalistic play activities (Phase 2) and activities within communicative and conversational contexts (Phase 3 and Phase 4).

- Before describing the specific phases of the treatment paradigm, the following aspects are important components in intervention:

  - It is important to ensure that the treatment stimuli are meaningful to the child. The child should be familiar with the vocabulary and pictured stimuli that are being utilized in intervention.

  - The contrastive pairs must remain paired in the early phases of intervention in order to draw the child's attention to the contrast being trained. Practicing each word in the pair separately will not draw the child's attention to the differences in meaning that are made by the change in his or her error production (that is, comparison sound) and the target sound.

  - It is important to use linguistic or communicative feedback to inform the child that there is a need for them to make a change in their productions in order to be understood. For example, in the contrastive pair of "Sue" ~ "two," the child says [tu] for both words. The clinician would provide linguistic feedback such as, "Is her name 'two'? That's silly! Her name is Sue!"

  - It is important to keep the activity moving and not drill on a given set of words in a contrastive pair. Provide the child with linguistic feedback following each pair, and then move on to the next pair. The child will have plenty of opportunities to learn the rule or contrast by going through the additional pairs that comprise the training set. Recall that the focused practice will result in around 60–100 responses in a 30-minute session.

- As shown in Figure 4–1, four treatment phases are incorporated in the paradigm, and treatment and generalization criteria are specified.
- With the exception of Phase 1, which is an introductory phase, movement to all subsequent phases or steps within a phase is data-based and driven by the child's performance. Three different criteria are established within the paradigm to govern movement throughout intervention and determine ultimate discontinuation of intervention on a particular target.

1. *Training criterion* is specified for Phase 2 and Phase 3 and steps within Phase 2.
   - The training criterion guides the clinician in making treatment decisions of when to move from imitation to spontaneous production and when to add additional treatment exemplars or move to more communicative contexts in treatment.
   - Specifically, the training criterion for changing from imitative to spontaneous production in Phase 2 is 70% accuracy across two consecutive training sets. A training set consists of 20 responses for minimal pair therapy and 20–50 responses for multiple oppositions, depending on the number of contrasts that are being trained. If five contrastive exemplars are used, a training set of 20 responses would be four presentations (or repetitions) of five minimal pair exemplars in a random order or two presentations of five multiple opposition exemplars of a three-way contrast (that is, [t] ~ [s, k]).
   - Once the training criterion is achieved at this level, intervention switches to spontaneous production. The new training criterion at this level is 90% accuracy across two consecutive training sets.

2. *Generalization criterion* specifies a predetermined level of performance that is required in order to judge that adequate phonologic learning has occurred and that no further intervention is required.
   - In the treatment paradigm, the generalization criterion is based on the child's performance on the target sound(s) in untrained items that are included on a generalization probe.
   - A generalization probe is constructed in which 10 words for each target sound in the trained position are included. The generalization criterion of 90% accuracy is used in the treatment paradigm.
   - Elbert and Rockman (1984) suggested that the generalization probe serves two purposes in intervention.
     - The more obvious purpose is to provide a measure of the child's learning of the target sound(s) in untrained items.
     - They also suggested that the probe can become a part of the therapeutic process, however, as the child begins to associate the sounds in training with the untrained items on the probe.
     - As a consequence of the dual purpose of the generalization probe, the child's probe performance might be inflated and not truly reflect rule acquisition.

3. *Criterion for discontinuation* is the final criterion specified in the treatment paradigm. In order to check the child's use of the target sound in conversational speech, a termination criterion is utilized.
   - Once the generalization criterion is met, a short conversational sample is obtained to examine the child's production of the new contrast in connected speech.

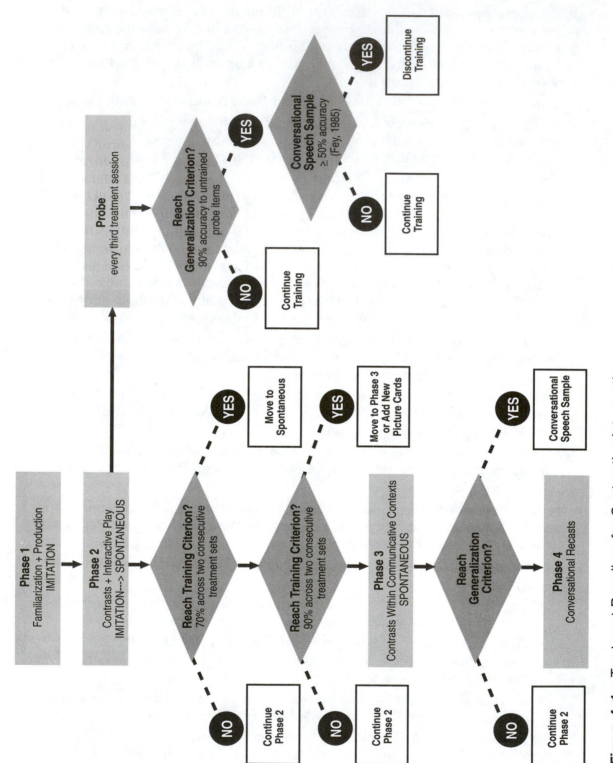

Figure 4–1 Treatment Paradigm for Contrastive Intervention

- Based on Fey's (1986) recommendation, if the child produces the sound with at least 50% accuracy in spontaneous connected speech, treatment for that sound is terminated.

Research Support

The number of treatment exemplars to be used in phonological intervention varies, and there is no set "magic" number that should be used. A study by Elbert, Powell, and Swartzlander (1991), however, examined the number of minimal pair exemplars that were needed for children to achieve response generalization to a larger, untrained set of items. Their results indicated that the majority of the children achieved generalization when trained with only three minimal pair exemplars. Although most children were able to achieve generalization on a small number of training items, the variability across the subjects was large.

There are four phases in the treatment paradigm. We will discuss each phase.

Phase 1: Familiarization + Production of Contrasts

- There are three steps to this phase:
  1. Familiarization of the rule that is being trained
  2. Familiarization of the vocabulary and pictured stimuli
  3. Production of the contrasts

Familiarization of the Rule

- Because rules are abstract and involve complex metalinguistic abilities to talk about them, it is important that the clinician make the rule "concrete" in order to make the rule meaningful and learnable to the child.
- This task can be done by making associations between the abstract rule and concrete examples of the rule.
  - For example, if the child is stopping fricatives and the rule that is being trained is frication, then the clinician can contrast "long" versus "short" sounds.
  - Tactile, auditory, and visual associations can be made for a variety of fricatives ("long sounds") and stops ("short sounds") in order to expose the child to the diversity and range of the rule.
  - The clinician could use crayons, markers, or chalk to draw long sounds on paper or on the chalkboard by making long looping lines as he or she produces and sustains different fricatives. Tactilely, the clinician could trace a long sound on his or her arm or the child's arm while producing a fricative.
  - Short sounds could be associated with making little dots on the paper while producing different stops. Tapping his or her finger on the arm or clapping the hands could be associated with short sounds.
  - Other examples for teaching some common rules to children include "open" versus "closed" or "empty" versus "full" for final consonant deletion; "tight" versus "loose" for gliding; and "things that go together" versus "something's missing" for cluster reduction.
- Familiarization of the rule should be a fun activity that involves active participation with the child. It should last approximately 10–15 minutes with repetition and redundancy of the concept. It will probably only require the first session to orient

the child to the rule that is being trained. The concepts introduced during this phase can be incorporated throughout intervention when instructing the child to use the "long sound."

Familiarization of Vocabulary and Stimuli

- It is important that the child be familiar with both the vocabulary items represented by the pictures as well as the pictures themselves. A child might be familiar with a particular vocabulary item but not with the stimuli in which it is depicted. For example, a child might be familiar with the word "see" but not be familiar with the picture that represents that word.

- One suggestion for familiarizing the child with the vocabulary is to tell a little story about each picture. For example, if the word is "fin," the clinician can explain that the fin helps the fish swim in the water. The fin can also be sharp and cut you. Then the clinician can ask if the child has ever seen a fin on a fish. This brief story about the word fin helps to put the word into a meaningful context for the child.

- Hodson and Paden (1983) suggest having the child draw his or her own interpretations of the training words as a way to familiarize the child with the vocabulary. Bonderman (1986) suggested using art projects in which the child creates his or her own stimuli for vocabulary items. For example, the child could paste a stem on a picture of a flower for the word "stem" or paint rocks for the word "rock."

- As a final step in familiarizing the child with the vocabulary and the stimuli, it is useful to go through all the contrasts as a review for the child. The clinician can place all the pairs on the table and play "teacher." The clinician will name the pictures and ask the child to point to the one named. This activity is not a test but a review, so it is useful to give clues to help reinforce the meaning associated with the pictured stimuli. An example is as follows: "'Straw.' I use a straw to drink a soda. Which one is 'straw'?"

Production of the Contrasts

- The final step of Phase 1 is the first time that the child has been required to produce any of the training items.

- The child begins intervention at an imitative level. The clinician provides an imitative model of both words in the contrastive pair and then asks the child to repeat the pair.

- Occasionally, this level of response of requiring the child to produce both words after the clinician model is too difficult. A branch step would be to produce each item of the pair and ask the child to directly imitate each word.

- Following the child's production of each minimal pair, the clinician provides linguistic feedback. This type of feedback is important in drawing the child's attention to the meaning in his or her productions. Linguistic feedback assists the child in eliminating homonymous productions and thus becoming a more effective communicator.

- Throughout intervention, it is important to create genuine communicative contexts as much as possible. In the early imitative phases of intervention, this goal is accomplished primarily through the linguistic feedback given to the child.

- In summary, Phase 1 is introductory and will generally only last for one to two sessions. This phase embeds the intervention in a meaningful context for the child. As such, the length of the phase is not based on data or the child's performance, per se. Rather, movement from this phase to the next phase is based on the child's familiarization with the training items.

Phase 2: Contrasts + Interactive Play

- Before discussing the steps involved in Phase 2, a comment about increasing the child's focus is important.

- As the child is learning the new rule you are training, it is important to keep training relatively simple without too many extraneous variables that will distract the child.

- Activities that involve playing board games or hiding the cards are too elaborate at this point for the child to effectively attend to the rule as well as to the production requirements of the individual treatment items.

- Such activities often result in a lower response rate from the child as well as a lower performance percentage.

- Keeping the activity simple at this point will help the child to focus on the new phonologic information. See "Analogy" for a nonclinical example of this principle.

- As in the "Analogy," the same principles apply to a child learning a new phonological pattern and articulatory routine. As the clinician, we must structure the intervention to allow the child to focus on learning the new contrast and rule. Gradually and systematically, we can admit those extraneous variables into the intervention process.

- As the child becomes more familiar with the rule, vocabulary, and contrast, more variety in the activities can be incorporated into intervention. Again, these variations do not have to be elaborate to keep the child's attention and motivation.

- It is amazing how simple variations to an intervention activity can keep the child's interest in the activity. Some suggestions for varying the activities include the following:

  - Place a chip, bean, or colored piece of macaroni on each pair as the child produces them.

  - Remove the chip from each pair as the child produces them.

  - Turn the pairs face down as the child names them.

  - Hide the contrastive pairs in a book and produce the name of the pairs as you turn the pages and find the pictures.

  - Toss the contrastive pairs into a large circle, container, or hula hoop as the child produces them.

  - Put a penny on each pair as the child produces them. The child repeats the pairs and this time keeps the pennies as he or she produces the pairs.

  - Hide the pairs around the room, and the child says them as he or she finds them.

  - Use an empty sprinkling can to water the contrastive pairs as they are produced.

Analogy

An analogy here might help clarify the importance of an increased focus at this early phase in intervention. A person learning to drive a car with a stick shift must attend initially to only the feel of the clutch as the accelerator is depressed. All extraneous variables, such as playing the radio, talking with other passengers, driving with one arm on the steering wheel, or applying makeup in the rearview mirror pull the driver's attention from the new learning task. These extraneous variables, however, can be incorporated later in the driving experience once the person is able to release the clutch and drive the car smoothly and automatically without thinking about when to release the clutch and when to depress the accelerator.

- During Phase 2, the child's accuracy rate will increase and his or her productions will become more stable.
- At this point, it is important to vary the order of presentation of the contrasts in each contrastive pair.
  - For example, randomly present the fricative first followed by the stop, and then present the stop item first followed by the fricative.
  - You might notice that the child's accuracy rate will drop when the presentation order of the pairs is varied.
  - This randomization will help the child learn the new contrastive rule rather than an articulatory routine.
- Often, children are in Phase 2, the longest of the four intervention phases of the treatment paradigm. It is here that the child is learning the articulatory requirements of the new contrast (imitation step) as well as the new phonologic rule (spontaneous step).
- There are two steps in Phase 2: imitation and spontaneous production of the contrasts.
  - The imitative step continues until the child reaches the training criterion of 70% accuracy across two consecutive treatment sets.
  - Once the training criterion is met, intervention shifts to the second step of Phase 2, which is spontaneous production of the contrasts. The training criterion changes to 90% accuracy across two consecutive treatment sets.
- Regardless of the steps in Phase 2, production of the contrasts occurs first, followed by naturalistic, interactive play activities.
- Phase 2 is similar to contrastive practice in Phase 1, with the exception that familiarization is no longer needed (and with the inclusion of interactive play of the target sound(s) at the end of the production practice.)
  - The purpose of the interactive play is to provide a more natural and communicative context in which the child is exposed to the rule that has been the focus of the treatment sets.
  - The interactive play provides opportunities for the child to practice his or her new contrast(s) during naturalistic play activities with a salient focus on the new rule.
  - It is hoped that the interactive play will provide a bridge for facilitating the child's discovery of the rule being trained as well as the transfer of his or her new productions in single words to connected speech.
  - This play period should focus on the rule that is being trained and provide several opportunities for the clinician to model and the child to attempt words with their target sounds.
  - Some suggestions for interactive play activities include the following:
    - "Bee, bee, bumblebee, I see something you don't see" is an activity that could be used for the child and clinician to take turns giving clues about objects in the room that have the child's target sound(s) in it.
    - Play house, have a tea party, play with a toy barn, plant flowers or seeds, look for leaves or rocks, go on an adventure hunt, use a craft activity, etcetera. Choose an activity that will have plenty of opportunities for the child to practice target sound(s) and for the clinician to model the target(s).
    - Read a book that has several words with the child's target sound(s). As you read, emphasize the child's target sounds and make them salient to the child.

Phase 3: Contrasts within Communicative Contexts

- Production of the contrastive oppositions and play are intertwined in Phase 3. The child plays games with the treatment exemplars.
  - Recall that the child moved from imitation to spontaneous at the end of Phase 2, so the child enters this phase at the spontaneous level.
  - In Phase 3, the clinician is able to be more innovative in creating more communicative contexts. At this level, the contrastive oppositions do not necessarily need to stay paired. The communicative activities will in themselves provide the contrast as the clinician responds to the child's meaning (see the following examples). It is often during Phase 3 that a child learns the new phonologic rule and achieves the generalization criterion.
  - Some suggestions for activities in Phase 3 include
    - Play Go Fish with the minimal pair cards. The clinician and client take turns drawing cards from one another in order to make a pair. During each turn, the person must ask for the matching card to make the contrastive pair. For example, the client might have all the open syllable cards while the clinician has the cards with the final consonants. The client has the card for "bee" and must ask the clinician for "beat."
    - Play classroom teacher by having the child tell the clinician to point to the card that he or she names. The clinician must point to the card named by the child, not the card intended by the child. This activity provides very strong communicative feedback to the child.
    - Play Concentration in which the cards are placed face down on the table. The child tries to match the pairs and say them as they are turned over.
    - Play What's Missing by putting the cards face up on the table. Have the child close his or her eyes while the clinician removes a card. The child then guesses which card is missing (Bonderman, 1986).

Phase 4: Conversational Recasts

- If the child achieves the training criterion at this point but has not obtained the generalization criterion, intervention switches to the conversational-based approach of naturalistic speech intelligibility training (Camarata, 1993; 1995).
  - At this point, the clinician recasts the child's error productions during naturalistic activities that are designed to provide frequent opportunities for the target(s) to occur.
  - The recast must be immediately contingent upon the child's errored production in order to make maximal use of hot spots, which are critical moments in which the child's awareness of and attention to the recast is optimal in utilizing the new contrasting information provided by the recast.
  - Activities are designed to have a high proportional frequency of occurrence of the new contrast in naturalistic activities.
    - Williams (2000b) reported on an activity used with a child who produced word-final /t/ and /tʃ/ as [k] in which the child was required to use the target sounds in a McDonalds restaurant scenario with the clinician.

- Menu items included a chocolate or peach doughnut, Sprite, carrot, and sandwich. The child needed to produce these targets in words to ask "How much is it?" or to complain when he found a roach in his sandwich.

- Many of the suggestions listed for the interactive play in Phase 2 can be utilized in this phase. Activities that will make the new phonologic contrast salient to the child should be used in intervention.

- Some suggested activities that can be adapted to the child's new rule include the following:
  - Craft activities
  - Adventure hunts
  - Making lunch or brownies
  - Playing in a sand box
  - Planting flowers or vegetable seeds

- The importance of the experiential activity is that the pattern is made more salient for the child by providing many opportunities for the clinician to model the new rule and for the child to produce the target(s).

- There must be a high frequency of occurrence of the target sound(s) in the activity that is developed.

- It is essential that the clinician keep in mind that it is not the activity that is important. Rather, it is the way the activity is used as a means to focus the new phonologic contrast(s) for the child in a conversational and play context.

- In summary, a treatment paradigm was presented that combined focused practice within communicative contexts while utilizing naturalistic play activities when appropriate.

- A series of phases and steps within phases were described with these main principles in mind.

- Generally, Phases 2 and 3 comprise the major part of the intervention program. Many children tend to reach training and generalization criteria by the end of Phase 3 and frequently do not require intervention in Phase 4. Refer to the following Research Support:

Research Support

Williams (2000b) reported on 10 children who received phonologic intervention using this treatment paradigm. Of these children, five children required conversational recasts intervention in Phase 4. Three of the five children were considered to have a profound phonological impairment (14%–29% of their sound systems were "known" relative to the adult system). The other two children who received training at this phase were in the moderate category of severity (54%–60% of their sound systems were "known" relative to the adult system). These two children were brothers who exhibited similar error patterns. It is difficult to determine from such a small N if intervention at a word level is sufficient for most children; however, there might be a tendency for children with greater phonological severity to need additional intervention beyond the word level.

LINGUISTIC PRINCIPLES OF INTERVENTION

WHO?   SLPs who work with children who have phonological disorders
WHAT? Linguistic principles that underlie phonemic models of intervention
WHY?   To understand the basis of phonemic models of intervention
HOW?   Utilizing the linguistic principle of contrasts to induce phonological change

- SLPs have incorporated linguistic approaches in their treatment of phonological disorders in children since the 1970s.

- Because different analysis frameworks incorporated linguistic principles and methodology in the description of speech disorders in children, it was consistent that treatment also incorporated linguistic principles in the treatment of the rule-based errors in children's sound systems.

- Before we discuss specific linguistic approaches, it might be useful to provide a brief discussion of the principles that underlie these approaches.

  - Starting with the basics, all languages of the world are made up of sounds, or phonemes, that are used to form meaningful words.

  - Speakers of the same language must learn these sounds that comprise the sound system of their language in order to converse with one another.

  - Phonemes serve a linguistic function in languages in that they *contrast*, or signal, a difference in meaning. An example would be words such as <u>p</u>at and <u>b</u>at or cu<u>p</u> and cu<u>b</u>. Each pair of words (pat ~ bat; cup ~ cub) has a different meaning that is signaled by the change of a single phoneme. Thus, phonemes are *contrastive*, and they function to distinguish meanings in a language.

  - Frequently, children with speech disorders *collapse* an ambient contrast, or distinction, that is present in the adult sound system. For example, a child who says [tu] for both "Sue" and "two" has collapsed the contrast between the adult phonemes /s/ and /t/. In this example, the meaning of the child's utterance is ambiguous. Does the child mean the person "Sue" or the number "two"?

  - The goal, then, of the SLP is to teach the child this phonemic contrast. This task is accomplished through the use of *contrastive therapy*.

  - The purpose of contrastive therapy is to induce a phonemic split by pairing the child's error production with the target sound in order to show that these two sounds signal a difference in meaning.

- As we will discuss in later sections, there are several different contrastive intervention approaches that differ with regard to the number of contrasts that are being trained and the type of contrastive pairs that are constructed.

- Regardless of the contrastive approach, all are conceptual and linguistic approaches by virtue of their emphasis on the meaning of what the child is saying, as well as to the new rule that the child needs to learn.

- Intervention is based on teaching the child a rule and not articulatory placement, per se. Consequently, a linguistic approach is *phonemic* rather than *phonetic*.

- In summary, linguistic treatment approaches address the function and use of contrastive sounds in the target, or ambient, language. When a phonemic contrast is absent (or collapsed), the goal of intervention is to induce a phonemic split through the use of contrastive therapy.

- There are several different contrastive approaches that employ aspects of the linguistic principles discussed. These phonemic models of intervention are listed as follows and discussed separately in the following sections:
  - Minimal pairs (Weiner, 1981)
  - Maximal oppositions (Gierut, 1989; 1990)
  - Treatment of the empty set (Gierut, 1990; 1992)
  - Multiple oppositions (Williams, 2000a; 2000b)

PHONEMIC MODEL OF INTERVENTION: MINIMAL PAIR THERAPY

WHO?	SLPs who work with children who have phonological disorders
WHAT?	Minimal Pair Therapy
WHY?	To eliminate homonymy
HOW?	Utilizing minimal contrastive pairs in phonologic intervention

- In the 1970s, assessment and intervention practices shifted from a sound-by-sound approach to a pattern approach. Speech disorders in children were viewed as a component of language and were therefore considered to be rule-based rather than peripheral motor problems. Grunwell (1987) summed up this perspective succinctly by stating that "phonological disorders arise more in the mind than in the mouth."

- According to Fey (1992), the goal of intervention is "to facilitate cognitive reorganization" of the child's sound system. Sounds are selected for intervention on the basis of their influence on other related sounds. Phonological intervention, then, is characterized by conceptual, rather than motoric, activities.

- Stoel-Gammon and Dunn (1985) stated that phonological intervention is ultimately aimed at generalization.

- One approach that has been demonstrated to accomplish this goal is minimal pair therapy.

  - Contrastive minimal pair therapy is the oldest and most common linguistic approach to phonological intervention (Ferrier and Davis, 1973; Weiner, 1981). This approach has been incorporated within various phonological assessment frameworks. It has been used with distinctive feature analyses (McReynolds and Bennett, 1972; Weiner and Bankson, 1978); phonological process analyses (Weiner, 1981); and generative analyses (Gierut, Elbert, and Dinnsen, 1987).

  - Minimal pair therapy is based on the notion of eliminating *homonymy* that results from the absence of an adult phonemic contrast. In this approach, the target sound is contrasted with the child's error production for that sound. The comparison sound is the child's error production and is specific to a given child's error pattern.

    - For example, minimal pair therapy for a child who produced [t] for target /ʃ/ would include contrastive minimal pairs, such as:

      "top" ~ "shop"   "two" ~ "shoe"

      "tip" ~ "ship"   "tack" ~ "shack"

    - In all these pairs, the child would produce both members of the pairs as homonyms. In these examples, the child would produce each pair as:

[tɑp]   [tu]
[tɪp]   [tæk]

- The goal of confronting the child directly with the homonymy would be to make them aware that in order to be understood, the child must change his or her productions.

- There are several published therapy materials for the contrastive minimal pair treatment approach. Commercial picture files are available that provide minimal pair cards for frequently occurring phonological processes, such as *Remediation of Common Phonological Processes* (Monahan-Broudy, 1991). Other materials, such as *Contrasts: The Use of Minimal Pairs in Articulation Training* (Elbert, Rockman, and Saltzman, 1980), contain picture files that can be used to make up any type of minimal pair treatment exemplars.

- Refer to the following Research Support for some studies that have reported the use of contrastive minimal pairs in the treatment of phonological disorders in children.

Research Support

Weiner (1981) reported a case study claiming that minimal pairs were efficient and effective in eliminating or reducing error patterns in children who displayed multiple phonological errors. Although a more recent study by Ingham and Saben (1991) questioned the effectiveness of minimal pair therapy, this approach has generally been widely adopted as a phonemic approach for children with speech disorders.

PHONEMIC MODEL OF PHONOLOGICAL INTERVENTION: MAXIMAL OPPOSITIONS

WHO?	SLPs who work with children who have phonological disorders
WHAT?	Maximal oppositions
WHY?	To facilitate phonological restructuring
HOW?	Utilizing maximal oppositions in phonologic intervention

- Gierut (1989; 1990) introduced a variation to the contrastive approach of minimal pair therapy, which she called "maximal oppositions." This treatment approach still contrasts two sounds, but there are important differences between maximal oppositions and minimal pair therapy.

- The major difference between the two approaches deals with the comparison sound that will be contrasted with the target sound. There are three criteria in the selection of the comparison sound that will be contrasted with the target sound:

    1. The comparison sound must be *independent* of the child's error. Recall that in minimal pair therapy, the comparison sound is the child's error production for the target. Using our previous example of the child who produces [t] for /ʃ/, the maximal opposition approach would select a different sound than /t/ to contrast with the target /ʃ/. The comparison sound would be selected on the basis of the following two criteria.

2. The comparison sound must be a sound that is produced *correctly* by the child.

3. The comparison sound must be *maximally distinct* from the target sound.

- Given these three criteria (independent, correct, and maximally distinct), the comparison sound in this example might be [m]. Contrastive pairs would then be constructed, such as:

"me" ~ "she"   "my" ~ "shy"

"Mack" ~ "shack"   "mall" ~ "shawl"

- Because the comparison sound is independent of the child's error, the resulting maximal oppositions will not be produced as homonyms by the child. Unlike the homonymous productions that would result from the minimal pairs, the child's productions of these maximal oppositions would be as follows:

[mi] ~ [ti]   [maɪ] ~ [taɪ]

[mæk] ~ [tæk]   [mɑl] ~ [tɑl]

- With maximal oppositions, the child maintains a phonemic contrast between the pairs of words, although it is not the same contrast as in adult speech.

- Consequently, the elimination of homonymy is not directly addressed in intervention but is left for the child to discover and eliminate on his or her own (Gierut, 1989). According to Gierut (1990), the child is indirectly taught to eliminate homonymy by exposing the child to maximally distinct forms that are "structurally and functionally equivalent" (p. 541). She further suggests that the difference between minimal pair therapy and maximal oppositions might be that maximal oppositions involve a very different learning process on the part of the child in achieving the same goal of eliminating homonymy.

- Development of maximal opposition contrastive treatment sets can be done by using any existing picture card files. There are no commercial treatment materials specifically designed for this intervention approach.

Research Support

The first investigation of the effectiveness of maximal oppositions in comparison to minimal pair therapy was examined by Gierut (1990) with three children who exhibited phonological disorders. She reported that the results indicated that maximal oppositions were more effective than minimal pair therapy in the improvement of trained sounds and the addition of more untrained sounds to the children's phonetic inventory.

PHONEMIC MODEL OF PHONOLOGIC INTERVENTION: TREATMENT OF THE EMPTY SET

WHO?	SLPs who work with children who have phonological disorders
WHAT?	Treatment of the empty set
WHY?	To facilitate phonological restructuring
HOW?	Utilizing treatment of the empty set in phonologic intervention

- Gierut (1991) developed another variation of contrastive therapy known as treatment of the empty set or treatment of the unknown set. This approach shares some similarities to maximal oppositions in that the paired words used in training are not produced as homonyms by the child.

- Different from the other contrastive approaches, however, is that *both* sounds that are contrasted are produced as errors by the child. As a consequence, the child receives intervention on two target sounds simultaneously, rather than on a single target sound.

- Returning to our previous example of the child who produces [t] for /ʃ/, contrastive pairs would be constructed to contrast the target /ʃ/ with another errored sound that was also maximally distinct from /ʃ/, such as /r/. This situation would result in treatment pairs such as:

| "ship" ~ "rip" | "Shane" ~ "rain" |
| "shake" ~ "rake" | "shoe" ~ "roo" |

- Assuming the child produced [w] for target /r/, the contrastive pairs would be produced by the child as follows:

| [tɪp] ~ [wɪp] | [ten] ~ [wen] |
| [tek] ~ [wek] | [tu] ~ [wu] |

- Again, notice that the pairs would not be produced as homonyms by the child because each target sound represents a different error production.

- As with the maximal opposition approach, no specific treatment materials have been developed for this approach. The contrastive treatment sets can be constructed with existing picture card files.

Research Support

Gierut (1991) examined the effectiveness of the treatment of the empty set in comparison to minimal pair therapy with three children who had phonological disorders. She found that treatment of the empty set resulted in greater phonological change than was obtained with minimal pair therapy. Gierut further claimed that treatment of the empty set resulted in the addition of more untrained sounds to the child's inventory than occurred following minimal pair therapy.

PHONEMIC MODEL OF INTERVENTION: MULTIPLE OPPOSITIONS

WHO?	SLPs who work with children who have phonological disorders
WHAT?	Multiple oppositions
WHY?	To eliminate homonymy and reduce or eliminate phoneme collapses
HOW?	Utilizing multiple oppositions in phonologic intervention

- Recently, Williams (2000a; 2000b) described another variation to contrastive therapy called multiple oppositions. This approach shares some similarities to minimal pair therapy.

- As in minimal pairs, the comparison sound is the child's error production for the target sound. Thus, homonymy is directly addressed in this approach, unlike the approaches of maximal oppositions and treatment of the empty set.

- A fundamental difference between multiple oppositions and minimal pairs involves the number of contrasts to be trained. Whereas minimal pair therapy trains a single opposition, multiple oppositions train several oppositions simultaneously from across an entire rule set.

- As noted previously, children with phonological disorders frequently collapse a phonemic contrast that is present in adult speech. Their collapse is often across several adult sounds. That is, the child might produce one sound for several different adult sounds. For example, a child might produce [t] for the adult sounds and sound combinations /s, k, tʃ, tr/, which represents a multiple phonemic collapse. This collapse is represented in the following diagram:

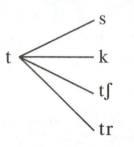

- Examples of multiple-opposition, contrastive sets for this collapse are listed here:

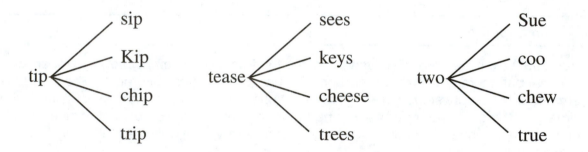

- The goal of multiple oppositions is to induce multiple phonemic splits rather than a single phonemic split as with minimal pair therapy. Further, the goal of eliminating homonymy will affect multiple homonymous forms in the child's speech. In the first example, the child would produce all the words "tip," "sip," "Kip," "chip," and "trip" as [tɪp].

- In this example, multiple oppositions would provide intervention across this rule set in order to eliminate the homonymy and induce multiple phonemic splits in this child's system.

- This approach maintains the child's rule set as an intact rule rather than a fragmented set of phonological processes that would label each of these substitutions with four different processes (stopping, fronting, deaffrication, and cluster reduction). Phonological processes miss the fact that the child's error comprises one rule rather than four different and unrelated rules.

- Williams (2000a) suggested that the learning of the "parts" of the rule, as in single opposition approaches, might negatively impact phonologic learning through the fragmentation of the new rule to be learned. Although learning distributed across an entire rule set can place additional demands on memory and attention, and increase semantic load, it appears that intervention that encompasses the whole rule contributes to the learnability of the new rule.

- The major concepts that underlie the multiple opposition approach are summarized in Table 4–1.

TABLE 4–1

Concept	Rationale	Specification
Part-Whole Learning	• Phonologic learning is facilitated by confronting the child with multiple error sounds from across an entire rule set, rather than addressing each error sound in a single, isolated contrast.	• Two to four target sounds are selected from a phoneme collapse and contrasted in multiple oppositions with the child's error.
Systemic (Re)Organization	• Phoneme collapses are viewed as compensatory strategies developed by the child to accommodate the full adult sound system with a limited, or restricted, child sound system. • The collapses typically reflect the child's attempt to "match" his or her limited sound system to the adult sound system along a particular phonetic dimension. For example, a child who collapses voiceless obstruents to [t] and voiced obstruents to [d] demonstrates an understanding of voicing and obstruent production. • As such, the phoneme collapses inform the SLP about what the child knows about the sound system and what he or she has yet to learn.	• Intervention is directed at phonological reorganization through the manipulation of the child's phoneme collapses. • The phoneme collapses become the means to an end in achieving phonological reorganization. • Targets are selected from the phoneme collapse according to a distance metric that has the potential to create the greatest amount of change in the least amount of time (see Systemic Target Selection Criteria).
Child-Based	• Intervention that is child-based—that is, directed to the child's phonologic strategies rather than an a priori set of rules or processes—will result in more efficient phonological change.	• Intervention is based on the elimination of phoneme collapses that exist in the child's phonological system. • Consequently, intervention is not based on predetermined phonological rules or processes.

Research Support

Williams and Kalbfleisch (2001) reported intervention data using the multiple opposition treatment approach with 14 children (mean age of 4 years, 9 months) who exhibited moderate to profound phonological impairments. They found that 86% (74/87) of the target sounds that were treated achieved statistical significance in 21 treatment sessions or less. Further, the majority of these sounds, that is, 74%, reached the spontaneous level of production by the end of the maximum of 21 treatment sessions. Finally, system-wide phonological change, as measured by productive phonological knowledge, significantly increased from a pre-treatment mean of 38.7% to a post-treatment mean of 62.5%. An increase was observed for each child.

- Supporting treatment materials for this intervention approach are currently being developed through a software program called *SCIP (Sound Contrasts in Phonology*; Williams, 2002). Although picture card files, such as *Contrasts: The Use of Minimal Pairs in Articulation Training* (Elbert, Rockman, and Saltzman, 1980) among others, can be used to construct the larger treatment sets of multiple oppositions, they are frequently time-consuming to use.

COMPARISON OF THE CONTRASTIVE APPROACHES

WHO?	SLPs who work with children who have phonological disorders
WHAT?	Contrastive phonological intervention approaches
WHY?	To select the most appropriate model of intervention for a given child
HOW?	Comparing phonemic contrastive approaches in terms of the number and nature of contrasts utilized in intervention

- Maximal oppositions and treatment of the empty set are similar with regard to the construction of contrastive pairs that are independent of the child's error and are maximally different from each other.
- To further understand the basis for these two approaches, let's return for a moment to feature geometry of non-linear phonology. By creating contrastive pairs that involve maximal differences in features that are high on the feature tree, such as [sonorant], as well as lower features of voice, place, and manner, feature geometry predicts that several new sounds will be added. This situation will occur because contrasts will be created at all tiers of the tree. Conversely, feature geometry would not predict the addition of several new sounds when the contrastive pairs involve only minimal distinctions that involve terminal features, which are lower on the feature tree.
- Gierut (1990) refers to the contrastive sound pairs in maximal oppositions and the empty set as "non-proportional." She states that non-proportional pairs do not share many features with other sound pairs. As a consequence of their uniqueness, the sound pairs are more salient and therefore more learnable. Compared to the proportional characteristics of sound pairs in minimal pair therapy, which share the same

features with many other sound pairs, Gierut suggests that learning the parts in proportional pairs might be easier but more difficult to place in the whole. Therefore, the saliency of non-proportional contrasts facilitates phonologic learning.

- How does the multiple-oppositions approach compare to the alternative contrastive approaches of maximal oppositions and treatment of the empty set?

  - Beyond the nature and size of the contrastive treatment sets, you will notice that the focus of the maximal oppositions and treatment of the empty set approaches is on the nature of the *sounds* being contrasted (that is, comparison sound ~ target sound for maximal oppositions; target sound ~ target sound for empty set). Specifically, sound pairs should be constructed to include non-proportional characteristics. It is predicted that increasing the saliency of the sound will therefore facilitate phonologic learning.

  - With multiple oppositions, the focus is on the *rule* and the *function* of the sounds within the rule. Specifically, sound pairs should be constructed to include sounds that represent extremes of the rule, or phoneme collapse. In other words, sounds are selected that represent the "corner pieces" of the rule, or puzzle. As such, the contrastive sound pairs are maximally distinct and might involve differences that are also non-proportional. It is predicted that learning will be enhanced through the increased saliency of the entire rule set.

  - The major principles of each of the four contrastive intervention approaches are summarized in Table 4–2. Each approach is compared according to several different parameters. As indicated in this table, the approaches that address homonymy directly (minimal pairs and multiple oppositions) share similarities, and the approaches that address homonymy indirectly (maximal oppositions and treatment of the empty set) are similar.

TABLE 4–2   Comparison of Contrastive Approaches

	Minimal Pairs (Weiner, 1981)	Maximal Opposition (Gierut, 1989; 1990)	Multiple Opposition (Williams, 2000)	Empty Set (Gierut, 1991)
Contrastive Pairs	error ~ target	correct ~ target	error ~ targets— phoneme collapse results in multiple contrasts	error ~ error
Contrastive Difference	Minimal or Maximal	Maximal	Maximal-Minimal	Maximal
Rationale	Eliminate homonymy by inducing a phonemic split	Increase phonemic distinctiveness to facilitate learnability	Eliminate homonymy and multiple phoneme collapses by inducing multiple phonemic splits	Increase phonemic distinctiveness to facilitate learnability
Severity	Mild-moderate	Severe	Severe	Severe
Approach	Linguistic	Linguistic	Linguistic	Linguistic

PHONEMIC MODEL OF INTERVENTION: CYCLES PHONOLOGICAL REMEDIATION APPROACH

WHO?   SLPs who work with children who have phonological speech disorders

WHAT?   Cycles Phonological Remediation Approach

WHY?   To present information on an alternative phonemic model of intervention, which does not involve contrastive word pairs

HOW?   Adapted from *Targeting Intelligible Speech* by Hodson and Paden (1983) and Hodson (1997)

- Hodson and Paden (1983, 1991) introduced the Cycles Phonological Remediation Approach, which involves a combination of traditional and linguistic approaches. Although it is a word-based approach, it does not involve the use of contrastive pairs.

- A primary feature of this intervention approach is targeting one of several selected phonological patterns within certain time periods called cycles.

  - A cycle is a treatment block of time generally ranging from 6 to 18 hours in which different targets across one or more error patterns are targeted.

  - For example, if the error pattern of final consonant deletion is selected for remediation, one-hour periods per cycle might be devoted to each specific final target, such as /p/, /t/, and /k/. Then a second error pattern, such as fronting, is selected with one-hour periods focusing on /k/ and /g/.

  - At the end of each cycle, the child's speech is reassessed and a conversational speech sample is collected. The reassessment provides information regarding the need to recycle the pattern or whether generalization to spontaneous speech has been achieved.

  - Typically, three to six cycles are required for intelligible speech to be achieved.

  - The treatment cycles are designed to reflect the child's natural acquisition process, rather than mastery of a specific target or pattern.

  - As noted earlier, production practice involves individual words rather than contrastive word pairs. Given the use of words rather than contrastive word pairs, Fey (1992) claimed that there was "nothing phonological" about the cycles approach.

- Hodson and Paden (1991) suggest that the selection of phonological patterns for the cycles approach should follow a developmental sequence, which begins with primary patterns, then secondary patterns, and finally moves to advanced patterns.

  - Primary patterns include early developing patterns that affect syllable structure, anterior/posterior contrasts, /s/ clusters, and liquids.

  - Secondary patterns typically involve palatals and other consonant clusters.

  - Advanced patterns focus on multisyllabic words with older children who have more difficulty at a conversational level.

- Another feature of the cycles approach is auditory bombardment.

  - The child listens to words that represent his or her target pattern for that cycle with slight amplification.

  - This activity is geared to "tune-up" the child's sound system in order to maximize the therapeutic input of the production practice.

- The principles that underlie the cycles phonological approach are adapted from Hodson (1997) and summarized in Table 4–3.

TABLE 4–3

Concept	Rationale	Specification
Cycles	Reflects the gradual nature of normal acquisition	• Error patterns are selected from Primary Patterns (syllable structure patterns, anterior/posterior contrasts, /s/ clusters, and liquids), Secondary Patterns (other clusters, palatals), or Advanced Patterns (multisyllabic words) • Specific sounds within an error pattern are targeted for about 1 hour per cycle • Several error patterns can be addressed within one cycle • One cycle lasts about 6 to 18 hours • The child's system is reassessed at the end of a cycle.
Auditory Bombardment	Acquisition occurs through listening	The child listens to 15-20 words through headphones at the beginning and end of each session.
Facilitating Contexts, Active Involvement, Self-Monitoring and Generalization	Phonologic learning is facilitated through the development of new kinesthetic and auditory images that occurs through production practice of words in facilitative phonetic contexts using a drill-play format. The new kinesthetic and auditory images that are internalized through production practice facilitate the child's self-monitoring skills.	• A small set of target words is practiced in each session using models and tactile cues. The goal is to help the child consistently produce the targets correctly in order to facilitate the new kinesthetic/auditory image. • 4–5 target words are drawn and labeled on index cards • The child actively participates in drill-play activities that last 7-8 minutes • A home program is developed in which the caregiver reads the auditory bombardment list of words to the child once a day and the child names the production word cards in a 2 minute/day home activity.
Optimal Match	Learning is facilitated by matching the child's current phonological level with an appropriate level in treatment.	Treatment is initiated at one step higher than the child's current phonological level in order to challenge the child while helping the child be successful.

- See the following Research Support for intervention studies using the cycles approach.

Research Support

Although the cycles approach has been used with children who have unintelligible speech and adapted for use with children with cleft palates (Hodson, Chin, Redmond, and Simpson, 1983), DAS (Hodson and Paden, 1983), and recurrent otitis media and hearing impairment (Gordon-Brannan, Hodson, and Wynne, 1992), there are no published data regarding the comparative effectiveness of this approach.

CONVERSATIONAL MODEL OF PHONOLOGICAL INTERVENTION: NATURALISTIC SPEECH INTELLIGIBILITY TRAINING

WHO?	SLPs who work with children who have phonological disorders
WHAT?	Naturalistic Speech Intelligibility Training (NSIT)
WHY?	To improve speech intelligibility in naturalistic intervention activities
HOW?	Utilizing a conversational based model in phonologic intervention

- Camarata (1993; 1995) introduced a conversation-based model of intervention called naturalistic speech intelligibility training (NSIT). This approach was developed to parallel the "naturalistic" movement in language intervention.

- Camarata (1995) made a case for more naturalistic phonologic intervention based on the following information:

  1. Many children with speech disorders do not display evidence of motor disabilities.

  2. Language and speech disabilities frequently co-occur in children.

  3. Speech disabilities are frequently associated with learning disabilities.

  4. Normal development does not include overt didactic drill activities.

- NSIT is based on Nelson's Rare Event Learning Mechanism (RELM), which includes growth recasts in which a new linguistic structure is embedded within a partial repetition of the child's prior utterance.

  - It was found that frequent presentations of growth recasts resulted in the rapid acquisition of new language structures. These exchanges resulted in "hot spots" where the child compares the stored "incorrect" form with the recently produced "correct" form.

- In the NSIT approach, clinicians recast the child's error productions without using imitative prompts or direct motor training.

  - Activities are designed to have a high proportional frequency of occurrence of the targeted sound in naturalistic activities.

  - For example, a child who is working on the sound [l] might play with Lincoln logs, Legos, lions, and other [l]-loaded items within a play activity.

- There are other conversation-based phonologic intervention approaches, most notably whole language (Hoffman, Norris, and Monjure, 1990). The impact of conversation-based approaches has been questioned (such as, Fey, Cleave, Ravida, Long, Dejmal, and Easton, 1994; Tyler and Sandoval, 1994), particularly with children who have phonological disabilities that are more involved than the small number of children who have been reported in the few conversation-based intervention studies that have been conducted.

Research Support

Camarata (1993) reported the treatment outcomes of two children using NSIT. The children, ages 3:10 and 4:3, were partially intelligible in spontaneous speech to family members and clinicians prior to intervention. The results of the study indicated that changes occurred in sounds with and without prior evidence of productivity. Further, the productions of both sound types generalized to spontaneous speech.

ARTICULATION (PHONETIC) MODELS OF INTERVENTION

WHO?	SLPs who work with children who have speech disorders
WHAT?	Models of intervention that are based on phonetic or motoric principles
WHY?	To improve the correct production of individual speech sounds
HOW?	Focusing on motoric positioning and movement of the articulators

- Traditional motor, or phonetic, approaches to intervention view speech disorders as a peripheral motor problem. Consequently, intervention was focused on the positioning and movement of the articulators.

- Just as there are different phonemic approaches (word-based contrastive approaches, cycles, and conversation-based approaches), there are several phonetic approaches available to the SLP who works with children with speech disorders.

- Although there are differences across phonetic approaches, there are many striking similarities.

- The most well-known and commonly used approach is Van Riper's traditional approach.

  - Although developed in 1930, it is still the most widely used approach today.

  - Variations to this approach did not appear until the 1960s with the McDonald Sensory-Motor Program (McDonald, 1964).

  - This variation was followed by several other variations introduced in the early to mid-70s.

- A summary of phonetic intervention approaches was adapted from Bernthal and Bankson (1998) and is presented in Table 4–4.

  - As we can note from this table, these approaches incorporate operant learning principles in the teaching of increasingly more complex motor skills as well as the use of a structured, contingent reinforcement paradigm.

- They differ primarily with regard to the specific structured sequence of steps included.
- It is interesting within a historical perspective to note that all of these phonetic approaches were developed prior to the introduction of linguistic principles in the form of phonological processes in the mid 1970s.
- Several of the approaches summarized in Table 4–4 will be described in the following sections.

PHONETIC MODEL OF INTERVENTION: TRADITIONAL APPROACH

WHO? SLPs who work with children who present with articulation errors due to impaired discrimination of speech sounds and/or inadequate development of articulatory skills

WHAT? Traditional articulation approach

WHY? To facilitate correct production of an errored sound(s)

HOW? Focusing on discrimination and motor training of individual speech sounds

- The traditional articulation intervention approach represents a compilation of treatment techniques by Van Riper (1939).
- This approach views speech disorders as a peripheral production difficulty that is related to auditory discrimination problems.
- Based on these assumptions about speech disorders, this approach utilizes "ear training" and a logical sequence of motor steps that involves drill on increasingly complex motor skills.
- The traditional approach is composed of five basic intervention stages:
    1. Discrimination or "ear training," which involves identification, stimulation, and discrimination of the target sound in isolation
    2. Sound establishment utilizing auditory, visual, and tactile cues
    3. Sound stabilization that involves drill on the target sound at increasingly complex linguistic levels: isolation, syllables, words, phrases, sentences, and conversation
    4. Transfer and carry-over activities that utilize speech assignments, self-monitoring, and practice in non-clinical environments
    5. Maintenance of the new sound through a gradual decrease in clinical contact moving from weekly sessions to monthly sessions and finally to sessions every three months, six months, and so on until dismissal from therapy
- The traditional approach has stood the test of time with numerous reports of improved speech intelligibility.
- Although this approach would not be effective for children whose speech errors are not motor-based or if their error patterns affect entire sound classes, many SLPs incorporate some aspects of the traditional approach in their intervention of speech disorders in children.

TABLE 4–4 Comparison of Articulation (Phonetic) Intervention Approaches

Approach	Assumptions	Features	Strengths	Limitations
Traditional Approach (Van Riper, 1930)	Discrimination problems are related to production problems. Drill on increasingly more complex motor skills.	"Ear training" Sequential motor steps embedded in increasingly more complex linguistic units	Most widely used approach Logical sequence of steps	Not effective for multiple sound errors or rule-based errors Vertical goal attack strategy is most often used, and this method is not efficacious for many children.
Multiple Phonemic Approach (McCabe and Bradley, 1975)	Sound errors are due to motor errors.	Structured format for data collection Structured sequence of tx steps Address several sounds each session (horizontal goal attack strategy).	Organized way to teach several sounds Data collection method	Not useful for group therapy Might be confusing for preschool children
Monterey Articulation Program (Baker and Ryan, 1971)	Sounds are learned motor behaviors. Contingent reinforcement increases desired behaviors.	"Recipe" step-by-step instructions	Good for clients needing high structured sequence in motor drill Good for instructional aids	Tedious
Stimulus Shift Articulation Program (McLean, 1970)	Generalization occurs through a systematic shifting of stimuli.	Treatment starts with words. Pairs and shifts stimuli to desired response	Pictured stimuli Small/systematic steps	All steps are not always necessary.
Paired-Stimuli Approach (Weston and Irwin, 1971)	Behavioral reinforcement paradigms facilitate the generalization from one context to others (stimulus-response generalization).	Pairing of words: Key word is paired with target words in which the target sound is not correctly produced	Builds on behaviors in child's repertoire Minimal time for instruction or directions High response rate	Need to train key word if child cannot produce sound correctly in a word

PHONETIC MODEL OF INTERVENTION:
MCDONALD'S SENSORY-MOTOR APPROACH

WHO?	SLPs who work with children who have articulation, or phonetic, sound errors
WHAT?	McDonald's Sensory Motor Approach
WHY?	To facilitate the correct production of an errored sound(s)
HOW?	Focusing on increasing the child's auditory, tactile, and proprioceptive awareness of the motor patterns of speech through motor production drills

- McDonald (1964) developed a sensorimotor approach to articulation intervention that was based on the following assumptions:

  1. The syllable is the basic unit of speech.

  2. Error sounds are produced correctly in some contexts.

  3. Phonetic contexts facilitate learning.

  4. Motor practice increases sensory awareness.

  5. The motor practice of syllables in different contexts and levels of complexity facilitates sound learning.

- Facilitative contexts are determined by administration of *The Deep Test of Articulation* (McDonald, 1964).

- Production drills are initiated with sounds that are produced correctly by the child in bisyllabic (CVCV) productions in which the vowel context and stress patterns are changed (for example, [pʌpʌ] with equal stress on the syllables, then produced with primary stress on the first syllable, followed by production with primary stress on the second syllable).

- Imitation of trisyllables is initiated that follows the same drill pattern used with bisyllables.

- The child is asked to describe the placement and movement of his or her articulators during the production of the bisyllables and trisyllables in order to increase sensory-motor awareness.

- Finally, the child produces the misarticulated sound in a facilitative phonetic context and drills on productions in various phonetic contexts in which the sound is not produced correctly.

  - For example, McDonald described the following treatment sequence for a child who correctly produced [s] in the context of "watchsun":

    1. Production of "watchsun" with equal stress on both syllables

    2. Production with primary stress on the first syllable

    3. Production of primary stress on the second syllable

    4. Prolongation of [s] in "watchsun"

    5. Production of short sentences (for example, "Watch, sun will burn you")

    6. Production of [s] in varied contexts (for example, "watch-sea", "watch-sit", and so on)

7. Production of [s] in other final [tʃ] contexts (such as, "teach-sand", "pitch-soon", and so on)

8. Production of [s] in phonetic contexts other than [tʃ] in which the rate of speech and the placement of syllable stress are varied

- Although some might consider a strength of this approach to be the initiation of treatment on behaviors that already exist in the child's repertoire, the bisyllabic and trisyllabic productions of nonerror sounds have not been shown to facilitate the correct production of error sounds.

PHONETIC MODEL OF INTERVENTION: PAIRED STIMULI APPROACH

WHO?	SLPs who work with children who present with multiple articulation disorders
WHAT?	Paired-stimuli approach
WHY?	To facilitate the correct production of individual sound errors
HOW?	Combining operant principles of learning theory with motor practice

- Irwin and Weston (1971) developed a highly structured approach to articulation intervention that begins at a word level and progresses to sentences and conversation.

- This approach utilizes operant principles in a behavioral reinforcement paradigm to facilitate generalization from one context to others (in other words, stimulus-response generalization).

- The primary feature of this approach is the pairing of a key word with training words.

  - Key words contain the target sound in words that are produced correctly by the child. A key word is one that the child produces correctly nine out of ten trials.

  - Training words contain the target sound in words that are produced incorrectly.

- Following the identification of a key word and selection of at least 10 training words, the following steps are incorporated:

  1. The key word and 10 training words are arranged on a picture board with the key word in the center, as shown here:

Sun	Seal	Soup
Sand		Soap
Sack	SEE	Suit
Sofa	Sandwich	Sue

2. Training begins with the child producing the key word and then one of the training words. The child is reinforced for the correct production of each word.

3. As the child progresses, he or she produces the key word: training word as a response unit, such as "SEE-Sun."

4. Subsequent steps involve production practice at the sentence level and in conversation.

- Specific goals and objectives, training criteria, and intervention steps and procedures are provided for each step and substep in the approach.

INTERVENTION ACTIVITIES: PHONETIC ESTABLISHMENT

WHO?	SLPs who work with children who have speech disorders
WHAT?	Facilitating techniques will be described to help establish the phonetic production of target sounds in the treatment.
WHY?	To help a child establish a new sound production
HOW?	Utilizing various facilitating techniques to establish the production of a new sound

Bleile (1995) categorized facilitating techniques for establishing a new sound contrast into (1) sound awareness activities and (2) direct instruction. We will discuss activities in each of these categories.

Sound Awareness Activities

- Three different types of activities can be used to help the child become aware of the new sound to be learned. These include (a) metaphors, (b) descriptions and demonstrations, and (c) touch cues.

- With each of these activities, the goal is to make the child aware of the sound(s) that is the focus of intervention. Another way of stating this description is to make something abstract, such as a sound, more concrete and meaningful to the child.

Metaphors

- Bleile (1995) provided extensive lists of metaphors for individual sounds (for example, [s] is the "hissing snake sound"), places of production (for example, "lip sounds" for bilabials or "biting sounds" for labiodentals), manners of production (for example, "long sounds" for fricatives or "nose sounds" for nasals), and for consonant clusters, syllables, and words (for example, "words with parts" for multisyllabic words or "sound friends" for consonant clusters).

Descriptions and Demonstrations

- Descriptions and demonstrations utilize different resources to demonstrate how a particular sound is produced.

- For example, using a tissue in front of the child's mouth to demonstrate the aspiration of the voiceless stop [p].

Touch Cues

- Finally, touch cues utilize tactile and spoken cues to facilitate the child's sound production.
- For example, place the child's finger in front of his or her lips for the production of [ʃ].

Direct Instruction Activities

- Direct instruction has been the cornerstone of speech therapy for decades. Although direct instruction is frequently associated with phonetic approaches to intervention, they certainly play a supplemental role within the phonemic intervention approaches, as well.
- There are two types of activities that can be used to help the child produce a new sound contrast: (a) phonetic placement cues (or moto-kinesthetic cues) and (b) shaping activities (or sound approximation activities).

Phonetic Placement Cues

- Phonetic placement focuses on the positioning and movement of the articulators.
- An example of a phonetic placement cue for the production of [f] is to ask the child to bite his or her lower lip and blow.

Shaping Cues

- Shaping uses a sound that the child can already produce, and through shaping techniques or successive approximation the child is gradually taught to produce a new sound.
- An example of a shaping technique for [s] is to start with the sound [t] and ask the child to rapidly repeat and prolong it at the end, producing [t-t-t-t-tsss].
- There are several resources for placement and shaping techniques. Bleile (1995) provides placement and shaping techniques for all American English consonants and vocalic [ɝ].
- As recommended by Bleile, these techniques should be reviewed and practiced in advance so that the clinician is familiar with the techniques and can adapt them accordingly with the needs of the child.

Other Facilitating Techniques

- Several additional facilitating techniques can be incorporated with the child to establish the new sound contrast to be learned. These include:
- Bombardment or flooding
  - For example, creating activities that include a high proportional frequency of the child's target sound, such as making a cage for your canary named Katie who eats carrots, cabbage, cookies, and candy. This method is similar to the naturalistic phonologic activities described under Phase 2 of the treatment paradigm.

- Facilitative talk:
  - Motherese:
    - Talking with exaggerated intonation and at a higher pitch; using short repetitive utterances (for example: "Oh, ball! See the ball. Big ball")
  - Expansions:
    - Repeating child's utterance and filling in missing information (for example, saying "Yes, boat" to the child's utterance of [bo])
  - Strategic errors ("confusion"):
    - Imitating a child's error production, such as [tu] for "Sue," to see whether the child notices the error and attempts to correct it. The classic response from a child is often, "Not [tu], [tu]!"
  - Parallel talk:
    - Commenting on the child's actions or play. For example, the clinician says "car" when the child reaches for the car and then might add "push car" as the child plays with the car.
  - Self-monitoring

"Tools of the Trade"

- As SLPs, we utilize several tools of the trade to facilitate a child's establishment of a new sound contrast by cueing the child for proper articulation placement.
- These tools include some of the following:
  - Tongue depressors (the new flavored depressors are popular with children)
  - Sterile gloves
  - Straws
  - Mirrors
  - Tissues
  - Diagrams, mouth puppets
  - Water
  - Peanut butter
- These tools should not be confused with the materials used in oral-motor exercises, which include icing, stroking, and strengthening exercises for the articulators.
- Most of these techniques have been borrowed from occupational therapy, particularly those involving sensory integration.
- Although these oral-motor practices are becoming more widely used by SLPs, there is a lack of evidence regarding the effectiveness of these techniques in facilitating sound production or the cognitive reorganization of phonological intervention.

Research Support

Forrest (2002) reviewed studies that examined the relationship between oral-motor exercises and speech production in children. Her review focused on three aspects of oral-motor speech intervention exercises: (1) transfer of training from simple non-speech activities to the highly complex and organized task of speech; (2) oral-motor exercises to improve articulatory muscle strength; and, (3) oral-motor exercises used to promote sensory-motor associations that serve as a foundation for speech acquisition. She concluded that oral-motor exercises cannot be considered a legitimate intervention approach for children who have phonological/articulatory disorders. Specifically, with regard to these three aspects of oral-motor training, Forrest summarized the following results:

(1) research has not demonstrated that training on part of the task increases the rate or accuracy of learning the whole;

(2) no experimental or descriptive studies provide consistent evidence that a strength deficit exists in children with phonological/articulatory disorders to warrant oral-motor exercises to increase articulator strength; and,

(3) oral-motor exercises cannot be used as a foundation for speech development since muscle activity for early behaviors, such as chewing, are distinct from the muscle activity involved in speech.

In conclusion, Forrest's review of the literature did not find evidence from empirical studies that support a facilitative or therapeutic relationship between nonspeech behaviors and speech production.

INTERVENTION ACTIVITIES: PHONEMIC INTEGRATION

WHO?	SLPs who work with children who have speech disorders
WHAT?	Activities that facilitate phonological restructuring through the phonemic integration of a new sound contrast
WHY?	To facilitate generalization and phonological restructuring
HOW?	Utilizing naturalistic and communication-centered activities

- Naturalistic and communication-centered activities help bridge the production of a new sound contrast within a limited treatment set of contrasts to an integrated, phonemic use of the new contrast within the child's sound system.
  - These activities are designed to facilitate the child's discovery of the new phonological rule. The interactive play provides opportunities for the child to practice his or her new phonological pattern during conversational play with a salient focus on the target pattern.
  - The activities should focus on the new rule being addressed and provide several opportunities for the clinician to model and the child to attempt words that contain the target sound.
  - These activities are similar to those described under Phase 2 of the treatment paradigm.
- One suggestion for naturalistic and communication-centered activities is to introduce the activity to the child and explain what sound(s) will be included.
  - For example, tell the child you are going to play Bee-bee-bumblebee and to listen for his or her "flat tire" sound.
  - This method helps link the activity back to the target sound and increase awareness of that sound. It might be too big a leap, particularly for a preschooler, to

pick up on a target sound during an interesting and fun activity even though you have developed a sound-loaded activity.

- Using the treatment paradigm described in a previous section, the naturalistic activities generally follow the completion of the focused production practice.
  - Typically, the clinician engages the child in a 5–10 minute naturalistic play activity.
  - During the activity, the clinician provides frequent and salient examples of the targeted sound(s).
  - The child's error productions are recast immediately following the child's production. For example, if the child says "I [ti] a [tu]," the clinician would recast the child's utterance by responding, "Yes, you did *see* a *shoe!*"
- Foils, protests, and setups can be used to increase the response rate, keep the activity going, and maintain the child's interest in the game.
  - Using the bee-bee-bumblebee activity, the clinician might take a turn pointing out something and mislabeling it (for example, "I see a turkey" while holding up a seashell). This method not only increases the response rate but can be wisely used in a competitive spirit to see who can identify the most items correctly.
- Typically, I prefer to use naturalistic activities initially that are more formulaic with higher response rates, such as bee-bee-bumblebee or other "seek and identify" type activities (such as treasure hunt, shopping, safari, grab bag, I Spy, Memory, and Bingo).
  - As the child progresses, the communicative nature of the activity increases while the structure of the activity decreases.
  - Later activities can include playing house, having a tea party, planting flowers or seeds, going on an adventure hunt, and making a craft.
- Generally, the naturalistic activities focus on one sound (for example, [s]) or one sound pattern (for example, fricatives [f, s, ʃ]).
  - If the child is working on multiple sound patterns or rules in intervention, I typically choose the sound or pattern that is the most difficult for the child.
  - Hopefully, this activity will provide an added "boost" to the focused practice that we complete for each session on that sound or pattern.

PROGRAMMING FOR GENERALIZATION

WHO?	SLPs who work with children who have speech disorders
WHAT?	A cognitive perspective of generalization
WHY?	To understand the construct and process of generalization in phonologic learning
HOW?	Incorporating generalization-enhancing activities into treatment itself

- Generalization has traditionally been viewed within a behavioral perspective.
  - Accordingly, generalization is viewed as a function of the stimulus properties and is primarily a passive process on the part of the child.

- Programming for generalization within this perspective involves a sufficient number of training exemplars and is viewed in terms of linguistic unit (for example, syllable, word, conversation), position (for example, word initial, medial, or final), or related sounds (for example, from one fricative to another).

- A cognitive perspective might be more appropriate within a phonological framework.

  - According to a cognitivist perspective, generalization is based on the child's available mental schemes and is viewed in terms of developmental change, such as category shift, category redefinition, and increase in category membership.

  - As "language engineers," we manipulate exemplars in ways that help the child make the necessary extraction and comparison processes occur in order to learn the new phonologic rule.

  - Therefore, explanations of change, or failure to change, are dependent on the resources of the learner *and* on the nature of his or her intervention experiences.

- The naturalistic and communication-centered activities discussed in the previous section fit within the cognitivist perspective of programming for generalization.

  - These activities provide new and wider patterns of phonologic use that are a composite function of what the child already knows and what he or she is able to induce from the language used by the clinician and the opportunities for practice that have been given to the child.

- In addition to the naturalistic activities that we can incorporate into our intervention sessions, we can also program generalizations into our intervention through the systematic manipulation of supports, prompts, and cues that we provide the child.

  - Initially, we provide maximum support to the child to increase the likelihood of being successful. There are numerous ways that we can boost the child's success. These might include:

    - We provide models that are salient acoustically and visually.

    - We supplement our models with physical cues (for example, running our finger down the child's arm as we produce a "long sound").

    - We might even shadow the child's production in order to provide additional support as he or she says the target word.

    - We control extraneous distractors in order to maximize the child's focus on the task.

  - As the child achieves success with our various supporting activities, we need to systematically withdraw these supports to provide learning opportunities to the child in more gradually difficult situations.

  - Culatta and Horn (1985) provided an excellent example of programming for generalization that incorporated this notion of the systematic reduction of supports. They suggested that generalization is programmed into our intervention activities through the increase of situational complexity, along with a decrease of modeling.

PARENT INVOLVEMENT

WHO?	SLPs who work with children who have speech disorders and the children's parents
WHAT?	Parent involvement programs
WHY?	To facilitate phonologic learning
HOW?	Incorporating parents in naturalistic home activities to facilitate learning and generalization

- Although there is a long history of incorporating parents in the intervention process, there was a revival of this practice in the 1980s as our caseloads increased and federal legislation (PL 99-457) mandated the incorporation of family-based practices.

- Several advantages have been reported for using parents as intervention partners:

  - Training parents as interventionists might be a time-saving process that facilitates the child's acquisition of a particular phonological target

  - Parental participation might ease frustration and anxiety by promoting parents' perceptions of themselves as a positive factor in their child's progress.

  - Parent-child interactions become "therapy" sessions within the home environment, thereby promoting generalization of new phonological contrasts.

- Fey (1986) stated that parents have typically been used in behaviorally oriented activities regardless of whether they assist the SLP as an aid or take responsibility as the primary intervention agent with their child.

- In the past couple of decades, there has been a shift away from behaviorally oriented activities to more naturalistic intervention home activities. This shift paralleled the move from trainer-oriented intervention programs to hybrid and child-oriented programs and emphasized the role that parents play in their child's development as natural language facilitators and interactors. See the accompanying Research Support at the end of this section.

- A parent-involvement program that I incorporate in the Phonology Intervention Program at East Tennessee State University utilizes naturalistic activities that families can do with their child during regular family routines.

  - The approach to parent involvement is based on three assumptions:

    - Learning is facilitated through naturalistic activities rather than through drill activities that involve practicing sets of sound cards or worksheets.

    - Time is limited for most families, many of whom are single-parent families or two wage-earner families.

    - Home activities that are developed within daily or typical family routines will be more likely implemented on a more regular basis and within more communication-centered activities.

  - This parent-involvement program, therefore, includes the following three components:

    - Parent interview to obtain information about a typical day and daily routines in which the parent and child (and siblings) are engaged

    - Developing home activities that are given to the parents each week to incorporate during their regular daily routine

- Follow-up on a weekly basis with a parent questionnaire to determine how successful the activities were and the amount of time and number of times that the parent and child carried out the activities within the week.
- These three components are described in Table 4–5.

TABLE 4–5

Parent Interview	Home Activities	Follow-Up

• A 20-30 minute interview is conducted to gain information about daily routines and a typical day for the parent and child (and siblings, if appropriate).
  • Information is obtained about morning routines (for example, who gets up first, does the child dress him/herself, breakfast routine, going to preschool/school, etc.); after school routines; dinner routines; bath routines; bedtime routines; and weekend routines.
  • The more information we obtain, and the more specific it is about the family's daily routines, the easier it is to design home activities that will fit into their regular schedule.
• The parent conference is also used to provide the parents with information about how children learn sounds and language.
  • Children acquire a sound system as active and creative learners in meaningful contexts
  • We facilitate learning through models that are salient and have an increased frequency of occurrence
	• Generally, two home activities are developed each week.
	• These activities are embedded within a particular daily routine, such as driving the child to preschool, grocery shopping, laundry, setting the table, bathtime, and so on.
	• Information is provided to the parent regarding the sound or pattern on which the activities are based.
	• A brief description is provided in writing for each home activity.
	• An example of a home activity is provided in the Clinical Example.
		• We establish a regular weekly schedule of getting feedback from the parent with the use of a parent questionnaire
		• Each week the parent returns the questionnaire as they get the next week's home activities.
		• The questionnaire provides the clinician with information regarding the success of the activity, the number of opportunities during the week that the activity was implemented, the amount of time spent on the activity each time, and any questions or problems that were encountered in implementing the activity.
		• We also occasionally ask the parent to tape record the activity. We can listen to the tape to determine if there are any suggestions needed to redirect or facilitate the parent's implementation of the activity.

Clinical Example of Home Activities

During your weekly grocery shopping, see who finds the most items in the store that begin with your child's target sound [k]. For example, corn, cucumber, can of beans, candy, Coke, cupcakes, cabbage, cauliflower, and so on. You can extend the game by using protests. For example, mistakenly label the "corn" as "tomatoes" and let your child correct you. You can also use protests with your child's labels. For example, if she identifies "candy," you can say, "That's not candy. That's spaghetti." Your child will have such fun correcting you, and you will elicit several target responses from her.

During bathtime, play a variation of "duck, duck, goose" that we will call "cat, cat, cow" to focus on your child's target [k] sound. With various toys in the tub, you each take turns touching a toy saying, "cat, cat, kitten." Whichever toy is touched on "kitten" is catapulted to the bottom of the tub. Using toys that start with the [k] sound will expand the number of target [k] models that your child will hear and produce (for example, cat, camel, car, key, cow, colt, cub, and so on). This activity might also expose your child to some new vocabulary words, such as "colt" for a young horse or "cub" for a young bear.

Research Support

Fazio and Williams (1986) investigated the effectiveness of parent involvement in language intervention with four preschool-aged children. Each child received intervention on two language goals. One goal received treatment in the clinic only while the second goal received clinic and home intervention. Children were matched on language goals with the order of treatment counterbalanced across children and "clinic only" versus "clinic + home." Results indicated that regardless of the specific language target or the order of training, children consistently demonstrated greater treatment and generalization performance on the "clinic + home" intervention goals.

SECTION

PHONOLOGICAL AWARENESS AND SPEECH DISORDERS

• •

This section includes information about phonological awareness skills in preschool-aged children. Information will be provided on the links among phonological awareness skills (or receptive phonology), speech disorders, and literacy. This section will conclude with information about the assessment and intervention of phonological awareness skills in preschoolers.

PHONOLOGICAL AWARENESS

WHO?	Speech-language pathologists who work with children with speech disorders
WHAT?	Receptive phonology, metaphonology, or phonological awareness skills
WHY?	To understand the relationships among the ability to manipulate sounds in a language, expressive phonological skills, and literacy
HOW?	Understand the relationship of phonological awareness skills to speech disorders and reading

- **What is phonological awareness?**

Phonological awareness skills refer to the explicit awareness of the sound structure of a language. This concept includes the awareness that words are composed of syllables and phonemes and that words can rhyme or begin and end with the same sound segment.

- **What is the link between phonological awareness skills and reading?**

Research indicates that phonological awareness is highly related to early reading ability. Beginning readers must gain a conscious awareness of the phonemes in words in order to learn to use an alphabetic language. Lack of awareness of sound structure makes it difficult to learn the grapheme-phoneme correspondence. This situation, in turn, results in poorly developed decoding and word recognition skills that are necessary for reading.

  - According to Blachman (1984), performance of phonological awareness skills by preschool, kindergarten, and first-grade children is a strong predictor of later reading achievement.

- **What is the link between phonological awareness abilities and speech disorders?**

Hodson (1998) reported that there is compelling evidence that children who have severe phonological impairments perform less well on phonological awareness tasks. Further, children with poor phonological awareness abilities experience greater difficulty learning to read (Stackhouse, 1997).

- **What is the importance of early identification of poor phonological awareness skills?**

The importance of early identification of deficits in phonological awareness skills was reported by Hodson (1998), who stated that time is a crucial priority given the critical age hypothesis that reading and spelling will progress normally if the intelligibility problem has been resolved by the age of 5 years, 6 months. Stanovich (1986) discussed the "Matthew effect" in which the speech impairments and reading difficulties are compounded over time such that "poor readers get poorer" and the "good readers" get better. According to Hodson (1998), unless intervention is appropriate and immediate, the gap between good and poor readers will widen over the years. Finally, Fey, Catts, and Larrivee (1995) note the importance of training phonological awareness skills as a crucial basic component of preschool language intervention in children with speech and language disorders as early as possible.

- **Can intervention improve phonological awareness skills and subsequently reading abilities?**

Blachman (1984) states that explicit training in phonological awareness skills has a positive and significant impact on reading and spelling skills. Further, phonological awareness training prior to a child's learning to read can be effective and have a subsequent positive impact on reading ability.

ASSESSMENT OF PHONOLOGICAL AWARENESS

WHO?	Speech-language pathologists who work with children who have speech disorders
WHAT?	Assessment of phonological awareness skills in preschoolers
WHY?	Performance on phonologic awareness tasks might have a predictive value for later reading difficulties.
HOW?	Through the use of several available standardized tests and nonstandardized tasks

- There are currently several commercial tests available to assess the phonological awareness skills of preschool-aged children.
- Some of the more commonly used tests include:
  - *Phonological Awareness Test* (Robertson and Salter, 1997)
  - *Phonological Awareness Profile* (Robertson and Salter, 1995)
  - *Test of Phonological Awareness* (Torgeson and Bryant, 1993)
- For older children:
  - *Comprehensive Test of Phonological Processing* (Wagner, Torgesen, and Rashotte, 1999)
  - *Lindamood Auditory Conceptualization Test* (Lindamood and Lindamood, 1971)
- These tests assess the child's ability to (1) segment words into their individual sounds, (2) identify and generate rhymes, (3) blend sounds, (4) categorize words based on initial and final sounds, and/or (5) delete or add sounds to make new words or break them down into syllables.
- In addition to these specific tests of phonological awareness, Catts (1997) suggests completing a battery of tests that assess additional areas that are frequently deficient in children who have poor phonological awareness skills.
  - Other areas that are often involved include word retrieval skills, verbal short-term memory abilities, speech production, and early reading and writing skills and knowledge.
  - Tests that can be used to examine these areas are listed as follows:

Word Retrieval

- *Clinical Evaluation of Language Fundamentals-3rd edition* (CELF-3; Semel, Wiig, Secord, 1995): confrontation naming subtest
- *Expressive One-Word Picture Vocabulary Test-Revised* (Gardner, 1990)
- *Test of Word Finding-2nd edition* (German, 1999)

Verbal Short-Term Memory

- *Token Test for Children* (DiSimoni, 1978)
- *Test of Language Development-Primary: 3rd edition* (TOLD-P:3; Newcomer and Hammill, 1997): sentence repetition

Writing/Reading

- *Test of Early Written Language-2nd edition* (Hresko, Herron, and Peak, 1996)
- *Test of Early Reading Ability-3rd edition* (Reid, Hresko, and Hammill, 2001)
- Catts (1997) has also published a checklist for teachers, as well as SLPs, to use to identify language-based reading disabilities. This checklist is reprinted in Appendix H, Early Identification of Language-Based Reading Disabilities: A Checklist.

TRAINING PHONOLOGICAL AWARENESS SKILLS

WHO?	Speech-language pathologists who work with preschool-aged children with poor phonological awareness skills
WHAT?	Remediation of poor phonological awareness skills
WHY?	Training in phonological awareness skills might facilitate reading and spelling abilities
HOW?	Through the use of various activities and commercial programs

- There are several domains of preliteracy knowledge, including phonological awareness skills.

- A framework for organizing the domains of preliteracy knowledge (van Kleeck, 1995; Adams, 1990) is outlined as follows:
  - The Orthographic Processor
    - Includes phoneme-grapheme correspondence, letter naming and recognition, and experience with print conventions
  - Phonological Processor
    - Includes phonological awareness skills such as rhyming and playing with speech sound units
  - Meaning Processor
    - Includes semantic, syntactic, and morpho-syntactic knowledge
  - Context Processor
    - Includes knowledge of book conventions, narratives, and expanded syntactic knowledge

- This framework is important in organizing the various intervention activities that can be incorporated in phonological awareness training.
  - Most intervention activities focus on the first domains, the orthographic processor and the phonological processor.
  - The latter two domains (meaning processor and context processor) are frequently addressed in language intervention activities that are not specifically directed at facilitating phonological awareness skills.
  - The intervention activities discussed for phonological awareness skills will be presented within this framework. Specifically, phoneme-grapheme correspondence, letter naming and recognition, and print awareness activities will be presented within the domain of the orthographic processor, and specific phonological awareness activities will be presented within the phonological processor domain.

Orthographic Processor Domain

- Letter naming and recognition involves learning to associate the shape of a particular letter with its name. This skill is a fundamental first step in learning to read, which requires the child to link the letter to the sound in sound-letter (or phoneme-grapheme) correspondences.

- Kamhi, Allen, and Catts (2001) claimed that the importance of letter identification has been overshadowed by the attention given to phonological awareness in recent years. Kamhi et al. further stated that the knowledge of letter names is as good a predictor of early reading ability as assessment of phonological awareness skills, if not better.

- A recent report from the National Reading Panel (2000) stressed that letters must be used in teaching phoneme awareness skills in order to help students make the phoneme-grapheme correspondence.

- Several activities are available to teach letter identification.
  - Examples of some activities are listed in the Clinical Activities box for letter identification.
  - Central to all of these activities is that they should be fun and enjoyable and avoid drills.
  - Also common to the activities is the incorporation of multisensory approaches. For example, have the child trace letters, feel them, write them, recognize them from an array of other letters, listen to their names, and say the names out loud.
  - The goal is for the child to be able to identify and name letters automatically. Many of these activities can be done at home by the parents.

- Given time and caseload constraints, what can SLPs do to facilitate letter identification?
  - Sound and letter recognition as well as phoneme-grapheme correspondence can be incorporated within regular speech intervention activities. Specifically,
    - The letters that correspond to the target sound(s) should be routinely present during articulation/phonological intervention. Write the name of the treatment words on each card. Make the target sound salient by writing it in red with the rest of the word written in black.
    - Utilize sound cards that represent the child's target treatment sound(s). For example, /s/ is represented by a picture of a car with a flat tire for the "flat tire sound." Place treatment cards next to sound cards in order for the child to associate the target sound with the picture and letter that represents the sound.
  - The SLP can also serve in one of three different roles:
    - Collaborative consultant, in which the SLP serves as an indirect service provider consulting with the classroom teacher to instruct him or her in letter naming and recognition activities
    - Planning team member, in which the SLP works as part of a planning team to design a language arts curriculum
    - Direct service provider, in which the SLP teaches or leads classroom activities for letter identification and phonological awareness

Clinical Activities for Letter Recognition
Kamhi et al. (2001) listed the following activities:

- Fishing for letters
- Identifying letters in books or worksheets
- Using letter-shaped cookie cutters with playdough
- Tracing letters in shaving cream, cornmeal, or sand

  Some additional home ideas/activities include:

- Use magnet letters on the refrigerator to make different words throughout the day/week; make family member names.
- Use foam letters for the bathtub.
- Use alphabet puzzles and alphabet sponge paints to provide additional opportunities for the child to experience and interact with letter names.
- Use alphabet cookie cutters to make cookies with family members' names or initials.
- Make alphabet pancakes; spell family members' names or make their first initial on top of the pancake.
- Read alphabet and sound alliteration books.

Suggested Alphabet/Alliteration Books
- *The Monster Book of ABC Sounds* (by Alan Snow)
- *An Amazing Alphabet* (by John Patience)
- *The Disappearing Alphabet* (by Richard Wilbur and David Diaz)
- *The Handmade Alphabet* (by Laura Rankin)
- *Aster Aardvark's Alphabet Adventures* (by Steven Kellogg)
- *On Market Street* (by Arnold Lobel and Anita Lobel)
- *Animalia* (by Graeme Base): an alphabet book of alliteration

Phonological Processor Domain

Catts (1991) categorized phonological awareness training into the following activities:

- Speech-sound awareness activities
  - Nursery rhymes
  - Finger plays
  - Songs
  - Rhyming stories
  - Stories with alliterations or with nonsense words
- Sound-play activities
  - Activities such as "sound of the day"
  - Developing a speech-sound collage

- Rhyme identification and production activities
  - Judging whether two words rhyme (example: Do "pan" and "fan" rhyme?)
  - Categorizing words according to rhyme (example: Find the word that does not belong)
  - Generating rhyming pairs of words (example: What rhymes with "hat"?)
- Segmentation/blending tasks
  - Breaking a word into its constituent sounds (example: [kæt] is comprised of three sounds: /k/, /æ/, and /t/)
  - Blending two or more sounds into a word (example: /p/, /æ/, and /n/ makes the word "pan")
- Sound manipulation tasks
  - Deletion activities (example: "cowboy" take away "boy" makes "cow")
  - Addition activities (example: /h/ plus "and" makes "hand")

Clinical Activities for Phonological Awareness

Roth and Baden (2001) listed several activities that promote early phonological awareness in preschool and kindergarten children. These activities can be used in groups, classrooms, or one-on-one intervention sessions.

- Songs, such as "The Name Game" (by Shirley Ellis), are a fun way to practice sound substitution skills with the names of different people or objects (for example, "Ali, Ali, Bo Bali, Banana Fanna Fo Fali, Fe Fi Mo Mali, Ali").

- Adapt the words to "Old MacDonald Had a Farm" to focus on different sounds. For example, "What's the sound that starts these words: *turtle, time,* and *tooth?* /t/'s the sound that starts these words: *turtle, time,* and *tooth.* With a /t/, /t/ here and a /t/, /t/ there, here a /t/, there a /t/, everywhere a /t/, /t/. /t/'s the sound that starts these words: *turtle, time,* and *tooth*" (taken from Yopp, 1992).

- SNAP game (by Burns, Griffin, and Snow, 1999) is played with one player saying two words. If the words rhyme (or share the same initial sound), the other player(s) say "snap" and snap their fingers. If the words don't rhyme (or share the same initial sound), the other player(s) remain quiet.

- "The Shopping Game" or "Sam Smith's Suitcase" are two activities to promote sound awareness using alliteration. In "The Shopping Game," the SLP names items purchased at the store that stress the initial sounds (for example, *cookies, candy,* and *carrots*), and the child(ren) generate other items that begin with the /k/ sound. The SLP can write the "shopping list" down to highlight the sound-letter correspondence. In "Sam Smith's Suitcase," the SLP says "I'm going on a trip and taking a suitcase. You can come too if you bring the right things." The child has to bring items that start with the same sound as his or her name; for example, Billy takes a bear, Billy takes boots, and Billy takes bananas.

- Catts (1991) provided the following reminders when training phonological awareness:
  - Phonological awareness activities vary in their cognitive and linguistic complexity.
    - Syllable awareness tasks are generally easier than phoneme awareness tasks.

- Continuant phonemes are easier to segment and blend than noncontinuant phonemes.
- Initial consonants are easier to segment and blend than final consonants.
- Tokens or blocks can be used to help in phoneme segmentation and manipulation tasks.
- Kamhi et al. (2001) also reported on the following guidelines from the National Reading Panel (2000) to teach phoneme awareness:
  - Focusing on one or two skills, such as sound blending and segmentation, is more effective than focusing on multiple skills.
  - Teaching phoneme awareness along with the accompanying letters is more effective than teaching phoneme awareness without the letters.
  - Teaching phoneme awareness is more effective in small groups than in either individual or classroom instruction. Furthermore, training programs that ranged from 5 to 18 hours of instruction were more effective than shorter or longer training programs.
- There are several commercial intervention materials available for phonological awareness. Some of the commonly used materials include:
  - *Sounds Abound Workbook* (Catts and Vartiainen, 1993)
  - *Phonological Awareness Companion* (Wellington County Board of Education, 1995)
  - *Sounds Abound Game* (Catts and Vartiainen, 1996)
  - *Phonological Awareness Kit* (Robertson and Salter, 1995)
  - *Earobics Auditory Development and Phonics Program Plus* (Wasowicz, 1998)
  - *Rode to the Code* (Blachman, Ball, Black, and Tanger, 2000)
  - *LiPs: Lindamood Phoneme Sequencing Program for Reading, Spelling, and Speech* (Lindamood and Lindamood, 1998)
  - *Seeing Stars: Symbol Imagery for Phonemic Awareness, Sight Words, and Spelling* (Bell, 1997)

Research Support

Gillon (2000) examined the effectiveness of phonological awareness intervention in 61 children (5 to 7 years old) who had phonological impairments. The children received intervention in one of three groups: (a) an integrated phonological awareness program; (b) a traditional intervention program that focused on improving speech and language skills; or (c) a minimal intervention program that involved consultation with the parents or teacher that focused on improving speech production skills. The results indicated that children who received phonological awareness intervention made significantly more improvement in their phonological awareness skills than children who received either of the other two treatments. Furthermore, children who received phonological awareness intervention also demonstrated more improvement in their spontaneous articulation of single words than children in the other two treatment groups. Gillon concluded that phonological awareness intervention might be an efficient approach to improving phonological awareness skills, reading development, and speech production skills in children who have phonological impairments.

A Final Research Note:

Recent research has examined the relationship between phonological disorders and phonological awareness skills in intervention. Specifically, will treatment of one aspect improve abilities in the other? Two recent studies have addressed this question from each perspective: phonological intervention and phonological awareness training.

- Major and Bernhardt (1998) found that phonological awareness skills improved following phonological intervention, although severity was a mediating factor. Specifically, children who had more severe phonological disorders required additional phonological awareness training to improve their skills in that area.

- In a reverse study, Adams, Nightingale, Hesketh, and Hall (2000) provided phonological awareness training and measured its impact on improving speech abilities in 31 children who had isolated phonological impairments. Their findings indicated that phonological awareness training resulted in significant improvements in speech output (as measured by PCC scores pre- and post intervention) as well as improved phonological awareness skills.

Obviously, this topic is an interesting and intriguing question that requires further study. Collectively, however, these studies indicated that there is a connection between receptive (such as phonological awareness) and expressive phonological abilities. As SLPs, we cannot ignore this important relationship in our assessments or interventions of children with speech disorders.

SECTION

INTERVENTION OUTCOMES AND TREATMENT EFFICACY

● ●

This section addresses the treatment efficacy of phonological intervention, measures for assessing treatment outcomes, and the use of single-subject designs in clinical practice. The final section will include a case study that will highlight these issues.

THE "THREE Es" OF TREATMENT EFFICACY

WHO?	Speech-language pathologists who need to demonstrate accountability for their clinical services
WHAT?	Assessing the efficacy of intervention in terms of effectiveness, effects, and efficiency
WHY?	To demonstrate accountability for our services
HOW?	Methods for evaluating the efficacy of treatment will be described.

- Olswang (1990) defined treatment efficacy in terms of the "Three Es": efficiency, effects, and effectiveness. We will now discuss these three components of treatment efficacy.

Efficiency

- Efficiency in intervention addresses two questions as a component of treatment efficacy.
  - One question deals with the length of time involved for the client to achieve goal(s).
  - The second question involves the amount of effort required to reach the goal.
  - Specifically, the questions for efficiency are
    - *how long did it take for the client to achieve his or her goal?*
    - *how much effort did it take to facilitate the observed changes?*
  - The first question, although simple to answer, is an important question. The number of treatment sessions that a client needed to achieve a goal provides an important context for interpreting treatment efficacy.
  - Each of two different treatment methods might have demonstrated significant improvement in the clients' performance. If one treatment method took 10 months to achieve the same goal that a second approach took only four months to accomplish, however, the two treatment approaches would be evaluated differently in terms of treatment efficacy.
  - Hodson (1998) suggested that all published treatment studies should specify the contact time with each child, including the number of sessions per week, the length of each session, and the period of treatment from beginning to end. She believes that this information needs to be included in order for readers to interpret the efficacy of the intervention.
- Other evidence that can be examined to assess the efficiency of intervention is a visual inspection of graphed data.
  - Specifically, is the slope of the client's learning curve flat, gradually rising, or sharply rising?
  - This measurement will indicate the client's progress in treatment and the length of time spent at different performance levels.
- The second efficiency question deals with the *amount of effort* required to obtain the desired goal.
  - We can answer this question by examining the child's response level in treatment and how long he or she remained at a particular treatment phase. For example, did the child remain at an imitative response level for a long time before moving to a spontaneous level?
  - Was there a need to include branching steps to help the child achieve his or her goal? For example, did the clinician need to incorporate simultaneous responding or use segmented productions for a period of time to facilitate the child's production of the new sound?
  - Finally, how much cueing did the child require to learn the new sound? Did the clinician need to use facilitative techniques or shaping procedures to help the child produce the sound correctly?

Effects

- Treatment effects address the significance of the observed changes. Specifically, *was the observed change significant?*
  - There are several types of evidence that help us determine the significance of the treatment effects.
    - Again, visual inspection of the graphed data (treatment and generalization performance) will provide information about the significance of the treatment effects. The slope of the graphed data will indicate the significance by a rising nature.
    - Pre-posttreatment measures can also be used to determine the significance of the treatment effects. Measures such as PCC, PCUR, intelligibility and severity indices, or rating scales can be compared for pre- and posttreatment to examine the extent of change following intervention.
    - Finally, we can use broader measures to evaluate "clinically significant" change. These measures might include conversational samples in which the child's production of the target sound(s) in spontaneous connected speech is examined.
      - Measures of social validation can also provide evidence of clinically significant change.
      - Questionnaires or rating scales can be administered to family members and teachers in order to obtain information from people other than the clinician regarding the significance of the changes in the child's speech intelligibility.
      - Using individuals who are not directly involved in the treatment is believed to provide a non-biased, objective measure that might not be possible from the treating clinician.
    - These broader measures and social validation measures are the ultimate test of the significance of the treatment effects.

Effectiveness

- Therapy effectiveness addresses the question, *"Was therapy responsible for the observed changes?"*
- The types of data that can answer this question include baseline level and trend, extended baseline, and control sound(s).
  - The level and trend of the baseline provide important information regarding the role of intervention in changing the child's performance.
    - If the level of the baseline is low (between 0–10%), then changes observed after the initiation of treatment can be attributed to treatment with more confidence.
    - Furthermore, if the trend of the baseline data is flat or falling (as opposed to a rising trend), greater confidence in the role of intervention in the observed change is gained.
  - Following from this discussion of level and trend of the baseline is an extended baseline.
    - Generally, a baseline period of three measures is recommended to assure a stable level of response prior to treatment.
    - If the baseline period is extended beyond this period (as in some of the experimental designs of single-subject research), then more certainty is attributed to the influence of treatment on the observed changes.

- Finally, using a control sound that does not receive treatment provides another source of evidence that change only occurred when treatment was initiated and was not a result of maturational factors.
- Gierut (1998) discussed the functional outcomes of published studies in phonological intervention by using the same "Three Es" of treatment efficacy.
  - The broader perspective of assessing treatment efficacy in published studies asked slightly different questions.
  - Specifically, the questions Gierut addressed with the "Three Es" are:
    1. Does treatment work?
       - Treatment effectiveness
    2. In what ways does treatment alter behavior?
       - Treatment effects
    3. Does one treatment work better than another?
       - Treatment efficiency
- Regarding question 1, Gierut (1998) stated that although there are different models of treatment available; these models can be categorized into sensory-motor and cognitive-linguistic approaches.
  - Different models within each category have been effective in creating phonologic change in children's sound systems.
  - The choice of which model to use in intervention follows directly from the diagnostic and classification framework that formed the basis of the SLP's initial phonological evaluation.
- The second question deals with the ways that treatment alters behavior. Gierut (1998) described different types of sound change to treated and untreated sounds.
  - Changes to treated sounds can occur across lexical items, phonetic contexts, linguistic units, and settings. We can measure treated sound changes by using specific (narrow) measures to trained sounds.
  - Changes to untreated sounds can be observed as within-class or across-class generalizations. Untreated sound changes can be measured by using general (broad) measures to untrained sounds as well as examine system-wide changes.
  - Two other measures of sound change include (a) online change to examine changes that occur during treatment and (b) longitudinal changes that examine change that occurs following intervention.
- The final question examines the efficiency of one treatment approach compared to another.
  - Gierut (1998) described three types of comparisons that can be examined with regard to efficiency:
    1. Comparison of different treatment models
       - The following comparisons have been examined experimentally:
         - Minimal pairs versus maximal oppositions
         - Minimal pairs versus treatment of the empty set
         - Minimal pairs versus cycles
         - Minimal pairs versus whole language

2. Comparison of types of sounds taught
   - The following comparisons of treated sounds have been made:
     - Early versus later developing sounds
     - Phonetically complex versus less phonetically complex sounds
     - Stimulable versus non-stimulable sounds
     - Most knowledge versus least knowledge
3. Comparison of modes of presentation
   - The following comparisons of modes of presentation have been examined:
     - Sound perception versus sound production
     - Drill versus drill/play versus play
     - Computerized instruction versus clinician instruction
- In summary, treatment efficacy encompasses three components that include efficiency, effects, and effectiveness.
  - Olswang (1990) and Gierut (1998) discussed each of these treatment efficacy components from slightly different perspectives and asked different questions within each of the components.
    - Olswang (1990) addressed treatment efficacy as a series of questions that a SLP can ask with regard to his or her own caseload and services to determine accountability.
    - Gierut (1998), on the other hand, addressed treatment efficacy from a broader perspective of what has been done in published treatment studies and what is known from the literature with regard to each of the three efficacy components.
    - A comparison of the questions asked by each are summarized in Table 6–1.

TABLE 6–1

	Olswang (1990)	*Gierut (1998)*
Effectiveness	Was therapy responsible for the observed changes?	Does treatment work?
Effects	Was the change significant?	What is the type and extent of sound change?
Efficiency	• How long did it take to achieve the goal? • How much effort was required to achieve the goal?	Does one treatment work better than another?

ASSESSING PHONOLOGICAL CHANGE

WHO? Speech-language pathologists who need to assess phonological change
WHAT? Qualitative and quantitative measures of phonological change
WHY? To identify and document change as a result of intervention
HOW? Methods for evaluating phonological change as a result of intervention

- Accountability and measures of treatment efficacy require clinicians to demonstrate the effectiveness of their interventions with clients.
  - Typically, clinicians rely on quantitative measures, such as percent accuracy, to illustrate a client's improvement as a result of treatment. Most of the time, quantitative measures capture the changes that occur in a child's sound system. A lack of quantitative change, however, does not necessarily indicate that no improvement has occurred.
  - The child might be making significant changes in his or her sound system that are not captured by "correct/incorrect" quantitative measures. Yet, these changes can also contribute to greater overall intelligibility.
    - Several researchers (Leonard and Brown, 1984; Rockman and Elbert, 1984; Weiner, 1981; Williams, 1993) have suggested that the extent of learning during intervention must also take into account qualitative changes.
    - Quantitative measures might miss the qualitative changes and the reorganization of a sound system that has occurred as a direct result of intervention.
- Qualitative procedures, such as phoneme collapses or Leonard and Brown's (1984) prototype model, provide a way to examine the child's integration of new phonologic information in restructuring their sound system.
  - These procedures require the clinician to examine the child's organization (via phoneme collapses or prototypes) in order to determine changes in that organization (in other words, reorganization) that occurs following intervention.
  - We will discuss each of these procedures as follows.

Phoneme Collapses

- Phoneme collapses involve a mapping of the child's system onto the adult's system. As noted previously, a characteristic of phonological impairment is a smaller sound inventory in relation to the adult inventory. As a consequence, there is a one-to-many correspondence between the child system and the adult system. This one-to-many correspondence is represented in the phoneme collapses.
  - A comparison of pre- and post-phoneme collapses can illustrate the phonological restructuring or reoganization that occurred as a result of intervention.
  - An example is taken from Williams (1993a) for a 6–year, 11-month-old child with a phonological impairment who demonstrated little to no quantitative improvement following intervention.
  - Examination of the following pre- and posttreatment phoneme collapses illustrates the reorganization that occurred, but it was not captured by quantitative measures.

Pre-Treatment   **Post-Treatment**

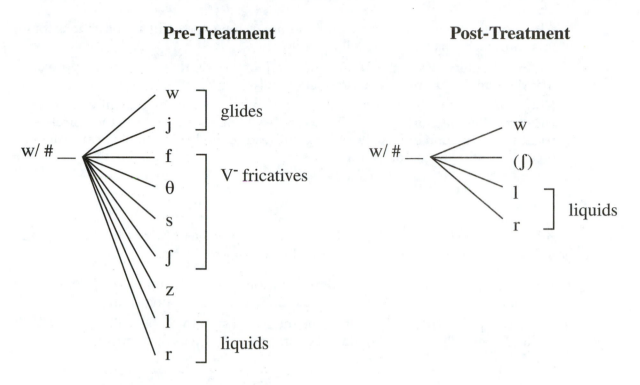

Note: ( ) denotes inconsistent correspondence

- Based on the pre-treatment collapse, the child received 13 45-minute intervention sessions that contrasted w ~ s / # ___.
  - As illustrated in these two phoneme collapses, the child actually exhibited significant improvement following intervention.
  - The reorganization that occurred was characterized by two changes: the number and range of sounds originally collapsed were restricted, and the collapses were more typical of developmental errors, such as the gliding of liquids.
  - Although the child quantitatively did not improve on his accuracy of target /s/ production following treatment, he added the fricative /f/ to his inventory and reorganized his sound system to incorporate this new sound.
  - His reorganization reflected a revised phonological structure, as illustrated in the new phoneme collapse that was present following treatment.

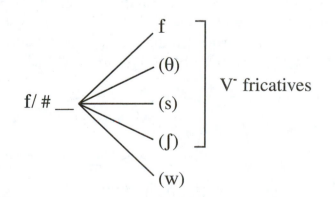

- Although the accuracy for target /s/ did not change, the child's productions for this sound did change as a result of treatment.

- Following intervention, the production of [f] for /s/ represents a closer approximation than his pre-treatment production of [w] for /s/.

- Notice that treatment on the voiceless fricative /s/ also resulted in all voiceless fricatives that were originally collapsed to [w] to be restructured to the voiceless fricative production of [f]. Thus, this child restructured his phonological system on a conceptualization of "fricativeness."

Prototype Model

Leonard and Brown (1984) described a child who expanded her set of word-final phonological possibilities based on a family structure resemblance, or prototype.

- Specifically, intervention facilitated the division and expansion of possible sounds to include new sounds that shared some similarities to existing sounds.

- Using this prototype model to describe the sound system of the child discussed earlier from Williams (1993a), the following prototype was developed:

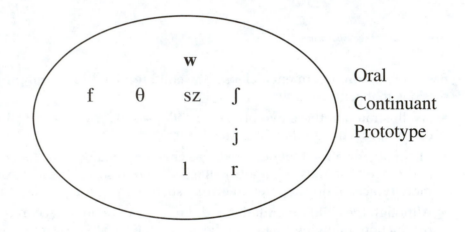

- According to the prototype model, the child's pretreatment phonological system is described in terms of an oral continuant prototype. Specifically, this child organized his system word-initially on the grounds of a family structure resemblance that was based on oral continuants.

- Intervention on w ~ s / # ___ facilitated the division and expansion of possible sounds to include new sounds that shared similarities to existing sounds.

- Specifically, the child incorporated the new sound, /f/, into his system. Consequently, his system was restructured, as illustrated:

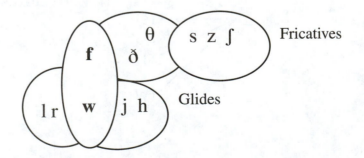

- The revised prototype illustrates the incorporation of a voiceless fricative (/f/) that created the phonological restructuring to break the glides and liquids away from the fricatives.

- In the reorganized sound system, the child produced fricatives for fricatives (primarily [f] for /s, z, ʃ/, but occasionally [θ] was produced for these sounds) and a glide for liquids. He also occasionally produced [f] for /w/, as represented by the overlapping circles that include these two sounds.

- Notice that these revised family resemblances share more similarities than the previous broad characteristics of being oral continuants.

- In summary, measures that incorporate qualitative aspects of sound change can provide previously undetected changes that occur as a result of intervention.

  - Qualitative information, such as that provided by phoneme collapses or prototype models, can provide clinicians with a window on children's phonologic learning, which reflects their active and creative hypothesis formulation and the organizing principles on which they structure their phonological systems.

USING SINGLE-SUBJECT DESIGNS IN CLINICAL PRACTICE

WHO?	Speech-language pathologists who are interested in the "practice of science" and the "science of practice"
WHAT?	Clinical research designs that can be used as tools to integrate the scientific method into clinical practice
WHY?	Two reasons: (1) to help the clinician be more efficient and effective in providing services to clients, and (2) to use as a tool to demonstrate accountability
HOW?	Several different single-subject designs can be incorporated in clinical intervention to allow SLPs to systematically evaluate and document patterns of change.

- Laney (1982) reported that increased demands on SLPs for accountability have created unprecedented needs for SLPs to become evaluators and researchers.

  - Others (c.f., Costello, 1979; Perkins, 1985) have pointed out the ethical responsibility of clinicians to question the efficacy of their treatment methods.

  - These two issues of accountability and ethics require clinicians to be both consumers and generators of research.

- One tool we can easily incorporate into our practice to generate research, as well as to demonstrate accountability and function ethically in our delivery of services, is the use of the applied research of single-subject designs.

  - Single-subject designs are tools that enable the research clinician or the clinical researcher to collect repeated observations or data about a client over a period of time.

  - These designs are "clinically based" and "practitioner-oriented" by their characteristics:

    1. They can be easily incorporated into clinical practice without disruption.

       - They can be used during regular clinical hours and during regularly scheduled intervention sessions.

- No control group is needed, so the clinician does not need to withhold treatment from a group of clients.
- The designs are flexible to allow changes during the course of treatment if the clinician determines that change is needed.
- Materials for recording and scoring behavior are no different than those typically used in intervention by the clinician.

2. Single-subject designs are "intervention designs."
  - Because they focus on individuals rather than on groups (as in research group designs), these designs can detect individual differences in response to treatment.
  - These designs gather repeated measures on a target behavior and therefore provide much more information about an individual's response to treatment than is available in pre-post measures.
  - These designs can be used to determine the effectiveness of a particular treatment approach.

- There are different types of single-subject designs.
  - The designs are typically designated by the letters "A" and "B."
  - "A" generally represents a baseline or no treatment period, and "B" represents a treatment phase.
  - Different single-subject designs are illustrated by the combinations and repetitions of the A and B phases.
  - McReynolds and Kearns (1983) described some single-subject designs that are listed in Table 6–2.

TABLE 6–2   Types of Single-Subject Designs

Phase(s)	Type of Study	Conditions of Study	Example
A	Descriptive	Baseline (BL) only (no treatment)	Diary study
B	Descriptive	Treatment (Tx) only (no baseline)	Case study
AB	Descriptive	BL + Tx	Case study
ABA	Experimental	BL + Tx + BL	Withdrawal or Reversal
ABAB	Experimental	BL + Tx + BL + Tx	Withdrawal or Reversal
AB AAB	Experimental	BL + Tx (behavior 1) BL^+ + Tx (behavior 2)	Multiple Baseline Designs • Across behaviors • Across subjects • Across settings

- Some points about these single-subject designs:
  - Notice that the first three designs are descriptive because there is no experimental control of extraneous variables.
    - A is a diary study (similar to the Hildegard diary study or the Brown diary study, in which aspects of the children's typical acquisition were documented).
    - B is a case study that can be used to describe the intervention of an interesting client. Limited information can be gained, however, regarding the effectiveness of intervention because there is no comparison to the client's behavior prior to treatment.
    - Although the AB design is another descriptive case study, it provides more information than the first two designs yet does not provide experimental control of extraneous variables.
  - The last three designs are experimental designs:
    - In the withdrawal or reversal designs (ABA or ABAB), there is a return to a no-treatment phase (A) after treatment has been initiated.
      - In the second A phase, treatment is withdrawn in a withdrawal design and the behavior should drop back toward the initial baseline level.
      - In a reversal design, the second A phase is used to introduce a behavior that is incompatible with the target behavior. For example, Elbert and McReynolds (1978) trained target /s/ in the B phase, and to reverse the behavior in the second A phase, they taught /θ/, which forced the behavior back to baseline performance.
      - These designs provide experimental control in that the scientific clinician or clinical scientist can demonstrate that treatment was responsible for the change in behavior and not maturation. This concept is demonstrated by the return of the target behavior to baseline levels in the second A phase by either a withdrawal or reversal of treatment.
  - There are three variations of the last experimental design. Each of these is listed here with an illustration:

(a) Multiple Baseline Across Behaviors Design

  - In this design, the same subject receives treatment on both behaviors.

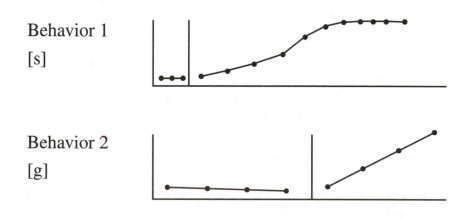

Behavior 1 [s]

Behavior 2 [g]

(b) Multiple Baseline Across Subjects Design

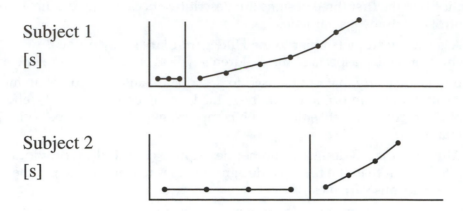

- In this design, each subject receives treatment on only one behavior, and the behavior is the same for both subjects.

(c) Multiple Baseline Across Settings Design

- In this design, one subject receives treatment on one behavior, but in two different settings.

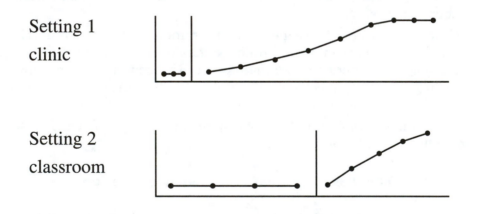

- Experimental control is demonstrated in each of these designs by a replication of treatment effects on another behavior, subject, or setting.
- The same treatment is applied to all behaviors, subjects, or settings in a sequence.
- Thus, the second behavior, subject, or setting serves as a replication for demonstrating treatment effectiveness.
- Williams (1993b) outlined five steps for clinicians to use single-subject designs in their clinical practice. These include:
  1. Define the behavior to be treated.
  2. Measure the behavior to establish baseline performance (generally three times prior to treatment).
  3. Select an appropriate design to evaluate the particular treatment approach to answer specific clinical questions.

4. Collect and graph data (treatment and/or generalization data).

5. Determine the effectiveness of treatment through a visual analysis of graphed data (trend, slope, and level of data points in baseline and within and between AB phases).

- In summary, single-subject designs provide a systematic tool for obtaining the accountability and ethical responsibilities in our clinical practices. Bloom and Fischer (1982) suggested that using these designs in intervention will make clinicians better practitioners as they approach their practice as a problem-solving experiment.

CASE STUDY

This case study presents longitudinal treatment data on the course of phonological intervention for a 4-year, 5-month-old child, whom we will call Eric, who was identified as exhibiting a functional phonological impairment that was characterized as severe to profound. Treatment was conducted over 19 months and included 78 treatment sessions. Eric's 19-month treatment history will provide information about the course of intervention as he progressed through the stages of clinically induced change to dismissal from treatment. Treatment efficacy will also be examined with regard to Olswang's (1990) "three Es" of treatment efficacy: efficiency, effects, and effectiveness.

Eric's medical and developmental history were unremarkable with the exception of severely delayed speech and language milestones. An oral mechanism examination revealed decreased lingual strength and range of motion.

Receptive language skills were assessed to be at age level; however, expressive language skills were impaired. From a conversational sample, Eric's MLU was calculated to be 4.17, and his utterances were characterized by frequent omissions of copula "is" (69%); auxiliary "have" and "has" (86%); and third-person singular (40%), as well as syntactic substitution errors involving irregular past tense verbs (50%).

Independent and relational phonological analyses were completed prior to intervention, at two points during treatment, and at the end of treatment. The initial phonological analysis indicated that Eric's sound system was characterized by only 14% correct, or adult-like, underlying representations. Conversely, 86% of his system was represented as "unknown" relative to the adult system. The predominant rules operating in Eric's system were phonotactic inventory constraints (71%) and positional constraints (15%). His limited phonetic inventory resulted in several extensive phoneme collapses, as diagrammed below.

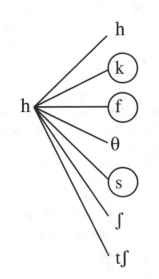

Word-initially, Eric collapsed voiceless fricatives and affricate to [h].

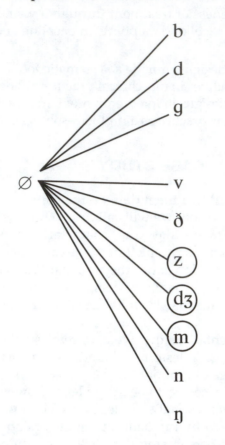

Word-finally, voiced consonants were collapsed to null.

Eric also collapsed voiced obstruents to [j] intervocalically, and voiceless obstruents were collapsed to a glottal stop post-vocalically.

In addition to the phonotactic inventory and positional constraints, Eric also demonstrated sequence constraints. For target clusters, he produced a singleton labial consonant, or [h]. Finally, labial assimilation was frequently present in the production of labial stops for alveolar and velar stops (and occasionally for [h]) in the context of round vowels.

In summary, the phonotactic inventory, positional, and sequence constraints severely limited Eric's phonetic repertoire and distribution of permissable sounds. This situation resulted in extensive phoneme collapses that greatly reduced his speech intelligibility.

Target sounds were selected on the basis of the phonological analysis and were indicated by the circled phonemes in the phoneme collapse. Specifically, target sounds were selected primarily on the basis of the function of the sound within Eric's sound system and secondarily on the basis of the distance metric.

Given the severity of Eric's phonological disorder and his extensive phoneme collapses, the multiple opposition treatment model (Williams, 2000) was incorporated in the initial phases of intervention. As Eric progressed in treatment, minimal pair therapy (cf., Weiner, 1981) and conversational recasts (Camarata, 1993) were incorporated. The structure of intervention (Fey, 1986) also changed as Eric progressed. Initially, the structure of intervention was horizontal and then moved to a cyclical structure.

Three measures were incorporated in treatment to assess treatment efficacy. Treatment data were collected during each session and graphed to assess daily treatment performance. Treatment criteria were established for determining progression in intervention according to the phonological treatment paradigm described by Williams (2000). Generalization data were also collected in order to measure learning on target sounds in untrained words. A generalization criterion was established for the termination of training. Finally, pre- and post-phonological analyses were compared to measure overall system-wide changes that occurred as a result of intervention. These measures are summarized in the following diagram:

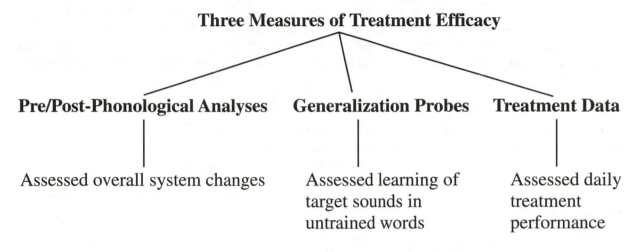

Three Measures of Treatment Efficacy

Pre/Post-Phonological Analyses | **Generalization Probes** | **Treatment Data**

Assessed overall system changes | Assessed learning of target sounds in untrained words | Assessed daily treatment performance

In addition to the phonological intervention that Eric received, expressive language goals were also addressed every semester of intervention. Furthermore, a battery of tests used to assess Eric's phonological awareness skills indicated poor phonological awaresss skills. Consequently, phonological awareness goals were also addressed every semester of intervention.

A summary of Eric's treatment goals and the intervention models is presented in Table 6–3.

TABLE 6–3. Treatment Models and Goals Across Semesters

Semester	# of Sessions	Treatment Model	Treatment Goals
Fall 1995	13	Multiple Oppositions	Ø ~ dʒ, m / ___# h ~ k, f / # ___
Spring 1996	18	Multiple Oppositions	Ø ~ b, m, n / ___# h ~ k, f, ʃ / # ___
Summer 1996	14	Multiple Oppositions	Ø ~ b, m / ___# h ~ k, f, ʃ / # ___ ʔ ~ p, t / ___ #
Fall 1996	18	Minimal Pairs	assimilation
		Multiple Oppositions	ʔ ~ t, k, f / ___ # h ~ t, k, f / # ___
Spring 1997	15	Minimal Pairs	assim d, g / # ___
		Conversational Recast	ʔ ~ t, z / V__V
		Minimal Pairs	t ~ tʃ / V___V s ~ st / # ___

Phonological treatment outcomes were examined with regard to Olswang's "Three Es." With regard to treatment efficacy, two questions were addressed:

- How long did it take to achieve treatment goals?
- How much effort did it take to facilitate changes?

Table 6–4 summarizes the answer to the first question. As indicated in this table, Eric significantly increased the proportion of his sound system that was "known" relative to the ambient system from 14% to 99% in only 19 months of intervention that involved a total of 78 treatment sessions. From Table 6–3, recall that Eric's treatment sessions incorporated three different treatment models and trained 13 different sounds across three word positions and one word-initial cluster.

TABLE 6–4. System-Wide Phonological Change Across Time

	Analysis I *(Sept. 95)*	*Analysis II* *(July 96)*	*Analysis III* *(Jan. 97)*	*Analysis IV* *(Apr. 97)*
Percent "known" relative to ambient system	14%	15%	88%	99%

[10 mo. / 1%]   [6 mo. / 73%]   [3 mo. / 11%]

———————— 85% increase ————————

(19 months /78 treatment sessions)

Thus, with regard to time efficiency, these data demonstrate that treatment was very efficient. This change is even more significant given the level of severity that Eric initially demonstrated.

Although intervention was efficient in terms of length of time, significant effort was required for Eric to make the changes that he did. As shown in Table 6–3, Eric received treatment on the same two error patterns, word-final collapse to null and word-initial collapse to [h] for three and four semesters, respectively. Furthermore, Eric required a simultaneous level of response initially in treatment before progressing to imitative and finally spontaneous levels of production.

Treatment effects addresses the question of whether the change was significant. Table 6–4 provides an answer to this question by comparing the phonological changes that occurred across the course of intervention. Notice that little to no change was observed following the first 10 months of intervention, yet significant change, 73%, occurred after the next six months of intervention, followed by another 11% improvement in the final three months of intervention. The change in Eric's sound system was significant, as shown by the total amount of improvement of an 85% increase in the "known" aspects of Eric's sound system in 19 months of treatment.

Finally, effectiveness was demonstrated by determining that treatment was responsible for the change observed in Eric's sound system. This result was demonstrated in two ways: (1) generalization to the target sounds in untrained words, and (2) no change in an untrained control sound that was included on the generalization probe.

The results from this case study provided information about the course of phonologic learning, which was important in evaluating the intervention program. These data indicated that initially there was little or no change in the child's system during the first 10 months of intervention, whereas there was an explosion in learning that occurred in the next six months of intervention.

There are two possible explanations for this pattern of learning. First, it might have taken additional time and intervention on the front end of treatment for the child to benefit from the therapeutic linguistic input provided to him, given the extremely limited amount of ambient knowledge he initially exhibited (14%). This account is similar to Elbert's "puzzle" analogy. Children who have fewer puzzle pieces require additional time to incorporate the new pieces of the puzzle to them via intervention.

Secondly, a motor component of learning appeared necessary for Eric to learn the new sound contrasts before learning a new phonemic rule. Recall that initially Eric required simultaneous and then imitative production in phonetically acquiring the new sound. Once the phonetic mastery was achieved, intervention focused on the phonemic use of the new contrasts at a spontaneous level of production. The interaction between phonetic and phonemic learning was discussed by Elbert (1992), in which phonologic learning might require both types of intervention by the clinician.

In conclusion, treatment efficacy was demonstrated in Eric's intervention with regard to efficiency, effects, and effectiveness. At the end of 19 months of intervention, Eric had eliminated the phonotactic inventory, positional, and sequence constraints that were present in his system during the initial phonological analysis. His phonetic inventory was complete, there were no gaps in his distribution of target sounds across word positions, and he produced consonant clusters. The remaining sound errors primarily involved occasional developmental errors on the sounds [θ, ð]. His overall speech intelligibility in connected speech dramatically improved with little or no difficulty in understanding his speech—even to unfamiliar listeners.

LIST OF APPENDICES

APPENDIX

PHONETICALLY REPRESENTATIVE WORDS ARRANGED BY PHONEME AND WORD POSITION

· ·

A. LYNN WILLIAMS
EAST TENNESSEE STATE UNIVERSITY

Phoneme	Initial	Medial	Final
t	tiger table teeth tongue	helicopter motorcycle octopus mustache	kite rabbit robot hat
d	dog dinosaur dove	birthday	red head
k	car cow/calf kite cake kangaroo comb	ice cream cone helicopter octopus Mickey Mouse	cake jack(s)
g	girl gum	wagon kangaroo tiger finger	dog pig
p	pig purple	purple apple Winnie the Pooh	jeep soap sheep
b	boy barn	rabbit robot table happy birthday	crab
h	house happy birthday head honey hat hands hay		
m	mustache motorcycle matches Mickey Mouse Marvin the Martian	ice cream cone umbrella Mickey Mouse Marvin the Martian	arm thumb comb gum lamb
n	nest	honey Winnie the Pooh dinosaur	barn ice cream cone lion queen sun violin xylophone green wagon van

Phoneme	Initial	Medial	Final
ŋ		finger kangaroo	tongue ring
f	fish finger	xylophone elephant	calf leaf rough
v	van violin	Marvin the Martian	dove
s	sun soap	ice cream cone glasses dinosaur mustache	house octopus jacks
z	xylophone zebra	present	nose ears eyes glasses hands matches
ʃ	shell sheep	Marvin the Martian	fish mustache
ð	this	feather Winnie the Pooh	smooth
θ	thumb three	happy birthday	teeth
tʃ	chair	matches	watch
dʒ	jeep jacks	object	orange
w	whale Winnie the Pooh wagon	pocket watch	
j	yo-yo Yellow	yo-yo	
l	lion leaf	elephant helicopter umbrella violin xylophone yellow	whale shell
r	rabbit robot red	arm motorcycle girl barn purple Marvin the Martian	tiger chair finger dinosaur feather

APPENDIX

COMMANDS INFORMAL ASSESSMENT

Name: _____   Date: _____

Examiner:_____

COMMANDS

Objects needed: baby, shoe, car, cup, and spoon

12 months

_____ Sit down   _____ Come here   _____ Clap hands

_____ Open door   _____ Open (your) mouth   _____ Stand up

_____ Where's object? (target response: looking behavior or other form of object recognition)

16 months

4-way object discrimination task to determine object recognition. Rearrange items after each trial.

_____ Touch / Where is / Show me baby.

_____ Touch / Where is / Show me shoe.

_____ Touch / Where is / Show me cup.

_____ Touch / Where is / Show me car.

_____ Touch / Where is / Show me spoon.

18 months

4-way object discrimination task. Rearrange items after each trial.

_____ Give me shoe.   _____ Throw shoe.

_____ Give me cup.   _____ Kiss car.

_____ Give baby kiss.   _____ Push cup.

_____ Give baby drink.

18–24 months

4- or 5-way discrimination task. Rearrange items after each trial.

_____ Put baby in shoe.

_____ Put shoe on floor.

_____ Give me car and spoon.   (or Give me car and give me spoon)

_____ Give me shoe and baby.   (or Give me shoe and give me baby)

_____ Push car and cup.   (or Push car and push cup)

_____ Throw spoon and baby.   (or Throw spoon and throw baby)

2–2$\frac{1}{2}$ Years

4- or 5-way discrimination task. Rearrange items after each trial.

_____ Put baby in shoe and give me car.

_____ Throw cup and push spoon.

_____ Kiss shoe and give me baby.

_____ Push car and put shoe on floor.

4$\frac{1}{2}$–5 Years

5-way discrimination task. Rearrange items after each trial.

_____ Throw cup, give me shoe, and kiss car.

_____ Put baby in shoe, push spoon, and give me car.

_____ Push car, give me cup, and put shoe on floor.

_____ Give me spoon, kiss shoe, and throw baby.

Gross Motor Commands

I.   _____ Show me (or "point to" or "touch") eye and mouth.

      _____ Show me (or "point to" or "touch") hair and nose.

II.   _____ Clap hands and open the door.

      _____ Stand up and close your eyes.

      _____ Bang table and touch your ear.

      _____ Jump up and down and touch hair.

III. _____ Open door, clap hands, and jump up and down.

      _____ Bang table, stand up, and touch ear.

      _____ Kick feet, open door, and come here.

      _____ Touch mouth, bang table, and kick feet.

APPENDIX

SYSTEMIC PHONOLOGICAL PROTOCOL (SPP)

A. LYNN WILLIAMS
EAST TENNESSEE STATE UNIVERSITY

#_

/p/	/b/	/t/	/d/	/k/	/g/	/f/	/v/	/θ/	/ð/	/s/	/z/
page	bathe	tack	do	cut	gain	fill	view	think	that	sing	zip
pages	bathing	tall	dive	cutting	go	fan	vote	thing	them	singing	zipper
path	bed	taller	diving	cook	going	fanning	voting	thirteen	they	sob	zoom
pig	beehive	teeth	doll	cookie	gauge	fog	valley	thumb	this	sobbing	zooming
piggy	behind	tongue	dolly	come	gauges	foggy	van		those	scissors	zombie
pay	buy	toothache	duck	coming	gush	fun	visit			seven	zero
pitch	big		ducky	catch	gushing	funny				south	
pitching	booth		dinosaur	catching	gum	father					
push	boss		donkey	cough	gun	feather					
pushing	bossy		doughnut	coughing		fudge					
python				kiss							
				kissing							
				coyote							
				Kathy							
				kayak							
				keyhole							

V_V

/p/	/b/	/t/	/d/	/k/	/g/	/f/	/v/	/θ/	/ð/	/s/	/z/
chopping	grabbing	retack	redo	recut	regain	refill	review	rethink	bathing	resing	rezip
hopping	robbing	eating	hiding	cookie	foggy	coughing	diving	Kathy	breathing	bossy	closing
shipping	rubbing	cutting	shadow	ducky	froggy	laughing	driving	Matthew	smoother	chasing	noses
zipper	sobbing	coyote	riding	quacking	hugging	sniffing	shaving	nothing	father	dressing	using
happy	strawberry	voting	reading	walking	piggy	elephant	heavy	python	feather	kissing	scissors
repay	rebuy	waiting	ladder	chicken	dragging		seven	toothache		dinosaur	sneezing
		thirteen									visit
		sweater									

_#

/p/	/b/	/t/	/d/	/k/	/g/	/f/	/v/	/θ/	/ð/	/s/	/z/
chop	grab	that	bed	kayak	big	giraffe	beehive	booth	bathe	this	bridges
hop	rob	eat	hide	cook	fog	cough	dive	cloth	breathe	boss	close
ship	rub	cut	rehide	duck	frog	laugh	drive	path	smooth	chase	nose
zip	sob	recut	ride	quack	hug	sniff	shave	south		dress	noses
reship	robe	vote	read	walk	pig	leaf	live	teeth		kiss	use
rezip		wait	reread	tack	drag		relive			yes	scissors
cheep		doughnut	tweed	retack	jug		glove			play-house	sneeze
rope		visit		magic			sleeve				gauges
				toothache							matches
											those
											pages

APPENDIX C   165

	/ʃ/	/tʃ/	/dʒ/	/m/	/n/	/ŋ/	/h/	/w/	/j/	/l/	/r/
#_	ship	charge	join	mail	nail		hide	wash	yoho	live	read
	shipping	charging	giraffe	mailing	nose		hiding	washing	yahoo	laugh	reread
	shave	chase	jelly	Mom	noses		hop	wait	yawn	laughing	reading
	shaving	chasing	Jimmy	Mommy	knee		hopping	waiting	yes	ladder	rain
	show	chop	jug	magic	nothing		hug	walk	you	lawyer	rainy
	showing	chopping		matches			hugging	walking	use	leaf	reach
	shower	cheep		Matthew			happy	watch	using	long	ride
	shadow	chicken					heavy	watching			riding
								wish			rob
								wishing			robbing
								witch			rub
											rubbing
											robe
											rope
											rebuy
											recharge
											recut
											redo
											refill
											regain
											rehide
											rejoin
											relive
											remail
											renail
											repay
											reship
											retack
											rethink
											review
											rewash
											rezip

V_V

/ʃ/	/tʃ/	/dʒ/	/m/	/n/	/ŋ/	/h/	/w/	/j/	/l/	/r/
reship	recharge	rejoin	remail	renail	singing	rehide	rewash	yoyo	relive	reread
pushing	catching	bridges	coming	fanning	donkey	behind	shower	coyote	dolly	stirring
crashing	pitching	guages	Mommy	funny	monkey	beehive	showing	kayak	mailing	scary
gushing	reaching	pages	blooming	rainy		keyhole	going	lawyer	taller	giraffe
wishing	watching	charging	zooming	dinosaur		playhouse	growing		elephant	strawberry
washing	matches	magic	Jimmy	doughnut		yahoo	throwing		jelly	zero
									valley	

#_

/ʃ/	/tʃ/	/dʒ/	/m/	/n/	/ŋ/	/h/	/w/	/j/	/l/	/r/
push	witch	fudge	gum	chicken	singing				keyhole	dinosaur
crash	catch	bridge	come	fan	sing				doll	stir
gush	pitch	gauge	Mom	fun	resing				mail	lawyer
wish	reach	page	bloom	rain	long				remail	scare
wash	watch	charge	zoom	gain	thing				tall	father
rewash			them	regain	tongue				fill	feather
			thumb	gun	nothing				refill	ladder
				join	bathing				nail	shower
				rejoin	blooming				renail	smoother
				python	breathing					sweater
				seven	catching					taller
				thirteen	charging					zipper
				van	chasing					
				yawn	chopping					
					closing					
					coming					
					coughing					
					crashing					
					cutting					
					diving					
					dragging					
					dressing					
					driving					
					eating					
					fanning					
					going					
					grabbing					
					growing					
					gushing					
					hiding					
					hopping					
					hugging					
					kissing					
					laughing					
					mailing					
					pitching					
					pushing					
					quacking					
					reaching					
					reading					
					riding					
					robbing					
					rubbing					
					shaving					
					shipping					
					showing					
					sneezing					
					sniffing					
					sobbing					
					stirring					
					throwing					
					using					
					voting					
					waiting					
					walking					
					washing					
					watching					
					wishing					
					zooming					

CLUSTERS

p + C	b + C	d + C	k + C	g + C	f + C	θ+ C	s + C	C + w	n + C/_#
playhouse	breathe	drive	crash	glove	frog	throwing	scare	quack	elephant
	breathing	driving	crashing	grab	froggy		scary	quacking	behind
	bridge	drag	close	grabbing			smooth	sweater	
	bridges	dragging	closing	growing			smoother	tweed	
	bloom	dress	quack				sneeze		
		dressing	quacking				sneezing		
			cloth				sniff		
							sniffing		
							stir		
							stirring		
							strawberry		
							sweater		
							sleeve		

APPENDIX

COMPARISON OF INTELLIGIBILITY MEASURES (KENT, MIOLO, AND BLOEDEL, 1994)

Procedure	Population	Sample	Measure
Phonetic Contrast Analysis			
CID Word SPINE; (Monsen, 1981)	HI children/ adolescents	written words	listener judges accuracy
CID Picture SPINE (Monsen, Moog, and Geers, 1988)	HI/deaf children	pictured words	listener judges accuracy
Ling Phonological Level Speech Evaluation; (Ling, 1976)	HI speakers	conversation	listener judges intelligibility (entirely ~ not)
Ling Phonetic Level Speech Evaluation; (Ling, 1976)	HI speakers	individual sounds/ syllables	listener judges consistency of production
Qualitative Rating of Performance (QRP); (Bross, 1992)	alaryngeal speakers	minimal pair words (I, M, F)	assess accuracy to derive QRP score
Speech Pattern Contrast Test (SPAC); (Boothroyd, 1985)	HI	phrases/ sentences	examine speech perception
Test of Children's Speech (TOCS); (Hodge, 1994)	preschoolers with motor speech difficulties	words/ sentences	assess accuracy
Children's Speech Intelligibility Test (CSIT); (Kent, Miolo, and Bloedel, 1992)	children with cognitive or motor limitations	words	listener judges accuracy
Phonological Analysis			
Assessment of Phonological Processes-Revised (APP-R); (Hodson and Paden, 1983)	children with phonological disorders	words	phonological deviancy score (PDS)
Functional Loss (FLOSS); (Leinonen-Davis, 1988)	children with phonological disorders	words or conversation	extent of homophony
The RULES Phonological Evaluation (RULES); (Webb and Duckett, 1990)	children with phonological disorders	words/ sentences	identification of phonological processes

Procedure	Population	Sample	Measure
Vihman-Greenlee Phonological Advance; (Vihman and Greenlee, 1987)	children with phonological disorders	large sample	Index of Phonological Advance (based on PP score, range of application score, frequency of application score)

Word-Level Intelligibility

Procedure	Population	Sample	Measure
Assessment of Intelligibility (AIDS); (Yorkston and Beukelman, 1981)	dysarthric adults	words/ sentences	number words correctly transcribed
Preschool Speech Intelligibility Measure (P-SIM); (Wilcox, Schooling, and Morris, 1991)	preschool children	words	listener judges from closed sets
Weiss Intelligibility Test (WIT); (Weiss, 1982)	children and adults	words/ conversation	1% words correctly identified 2% words correctly understood

Continuous Speech Intelligibility

Procedure	Population	Sample	Measure
Percentage of Consonants Correct (PCC); (Shriberg and Kwiatkowski, 1982)	unrestricted, but generally children with phonological disorders	conversation	Percentage of consonants produced correctly
Articulation Competence Index (ACI); (Shriberg, 1993)	unrestricted, but generally children with phonological disorders	conversation	PCC + RDI divided by 2 RDI=Relative Distortion Index

Scaling Methods

Procedure	Population	Sample	Measure
Meaningful Use of Speech Scale (MUSS); (Osberger, 1992)	HI	everyday speaking situations	parent/teacher report of frequency of behaviors
NTID Rating Scale; (Schiavetti, 1992)	HI	conversation/ reading	listener scores intelligibility on 5-point scale

HI = hearing impaired

APPENDIX

NON-STANDARDIZED PHONOLOGICAL PROCESS ANALYSIS SUMMARY SHEET

A. LYNN WILLIAMS
EAST TENNESSEE STATE UNIVERSITY

Client:_____ Date: _____

Clinician: _____ Age: _____

	FREQUENCY OF OCCURRENCE # TIMES OCCURRED # OPPORTUNITIES	AGE OF SUPPRESSION
Structural Processes (Deletion)		
Final Consonant Deletion (FCD)	_____	_____
Initial Consonant Deletion (ICD)	_____	_____
Cluster Reduction (CR)	_____	_____
Weak Syllable Deletion (WSD)	_____	_____
Consonant Deletion (CD)	_____	_____
Reduplication (RD)	_____	_____
Assimilation		
Labial Assimilation (LA)	_____	_____
Nasal Assimilation (NA)	_____	_____
Velar Assimilation (VA)	_____	_____
Consonant Harmony (CH)	_____	_____
Simplification Processes (Substitution)		
Stopping (ST)	_____	_____
Fronting (FR)	_____	_____
Gliding (GL)	_____	_____
Vocalization (VO)	_____	_____
Deaffrication (DA)	_____	_____
Apicalization (AP)	_____	_____
Labalization (LB)	_____	_____
Denasalization (DN)	_____	_____
Glottal Replacement (GR)	_____	_____
Palatalization (PL)	_____	_____
Voicing (Voi)	_____	_____
Devoicing (DV)	_____	_____

	FREQUENCY OF OCCURRENCE **# TIMES OCCURRED** # OPPORTUNITIES	AGE OF SUPPRESSION
Other Processes		
Idiosyncratic Processes (IP)	_____	_____
Other	_____	_____

Summary

Classes of sounds/positions affected by processes:

Consistency of processes:

Process interactions:

Persisting Normal Processes:

Idiosyncratic Processes:

APPENDIX

F

PLACE-VOICE-MANNER ERROR PATTERN ANALYSIS

Name: _____

Date: _____

Transcriber: _____

	Nasals			Stops						Fricatives										Affricates		Liquids		Glides	
	m	n	ŋ	p	b	t	d	k	g	θ	ð	f	v	s	z	ʃ	ʒ	h	tʃ	dʒ	l	r	w	j
Pre-vocalic #_																									
Inter-vocalic V_V																									
Post-vocalic _#																									

Nasal clusters	/l/ clusters	/r/ clusters	/w/ clusters	/s/ clusters	Phonetic Inventory	P.V.M. Error Patterns
nt · nd · ndʒ · mp	pl · bl · kl · gl · fl · sl	pr · br · tr · dr · kr · gr · fr · ʃr · θr	tw · dw · kw · gw · sw	sm · sn · sp · st · sk		

APPENDIX

SYSTEMIC PHONOLOGICAL ANALYSIS OF CHILD SPEECH (SPACS)

· ·

A. LYNN WILLIAMS
EAST TENNESSEE STATE UNIVERSITY

Client: _____   Date: _____

Clinician: _____   Age: _____

PHONETIC INVENTORY (SYSTEMIC)

	Word-Initial	*Word-Final*
Stops		
Nasals		
Fricatives		
Affricates		
Glides		
Liquids		

DISTRIBUTION OF SOUNDS (STRUCTURAL)

	#_	V_V	_#		#_	V_V	_#
Stops p b t d k g				Affricates tʃ dʒ			
				Nasals m n ŋ			
Fricatives f v θ ð s z ʃ				Glides w j h			
				Liquids l r			

<u>Clusters:</u>

MAPPING CHILD-TO-ADULT SYSTEMS (PHONEME COLLAPSES)

Word-Initial #_	Word-Medial V_V	Word-Final _#

APPENDIX

EARLY IDENTIFICATION OF LANGUAGE-BASED READING DISABILITIES: A CHECKLIST

HUGH W. CATTS
UNIVERSITY OF KANSAS

SPEECH SOUND AWARENESS

☐ Doesn't understand and enjoy rhymes

☐ Doesn't easily recognize that words may begin with the same sound

☐ Has difficulty counting the syllables in spoken words

☐ Has problem clapping hands or tapping feet in rhythm with songs and/or rhymes

☐ Demonstrates problems learning sound-letter correspondences

WORD RETRIEVAL

☐ Has difficulty retrieving a specific word (for example, calls a sheep a "goat" or says "you know, a woolly animal")

☐ Shows poor memory for classmates' names

☐ Speech is hesitant, filled with pauses or vocalizations (for example, "um," "you know")

☐ Frequently uses words lacking specificity (such as "stuff," "thing," "what you call it")

☐ Has a problem remembering/retrieving verbal sequences (for example, days of the week, alphabet)

VERBAL MEMORY

☐ Has difficulty remembering instructions or directions

☐ Shows problems learning names of people or places

☐ Has difficulty remembering the words to songs or poems

☐ Has problems learning a second language

SPEECH PRODUCTION/PERCEPTION

☐ Has problems saying common words with difficult sound patterns (such as animal, cinnamon, specific)

☐ Mishears and subsequently mispronounces words or names

☐ Confuses a similar sounding word with another word (for example, saying "The Entire State Building is in New York")

☐ Combines sound patterns or similar words (such as saying "escavator" for escalator)

☐ Shows frequent slips of the tongue (for example, saying "brue blush" for blue brush)

☐ Has difficulty with tongue twisters (such as "she sells seashells")

COMPREHENSION

☐ Only responds to part of a multiple element request or instruction

☐ Requests multiple repetitions of instructions/directions with little improvement in comprehension

☐ Relies too much on context to understand what is said

☐ Has difficulty understanding questions

☐ Fails to understand age-appropriate stories

☐ Has difficulty making inferences, predicting outcomes, drawing conclusions

☐ Lacks understanding of spatial terms such as left-right, front-back

EXPRESSIVE LANGUAGE

☐ Talks in short sentences

☐ Makes errors in grammar (for example, "he goed to the store" or "me want that")

☐ Lacks variety in vocabulary (such as using "good" to mean happy, kind, polite)

☐ Has difficulty giving directions or explanations (for example, may show multiple revisions or dead ends)

☐ Relates stories or events in a disorganized or incomplete manner

☐ May have much to say, but provides little specific detail

☐ Has difficulty with the rules of conversation, such as turn taking, staying on topic, or indicating when he/she does not understand

OTHER IMPORTANT FACTORS

☐ Has a prior history of problems in language comprehension and/or production

☐ Has a family history of spoken or written language problems

☐ Has limited exposure to literacy in the home

☐ Lacks interest in books and shared reading activities

☐ Does not engage readily in pretend play

COMMENTS:

GLOSSARY

· ·

Ambient Sound System—the sound system of the surrounding, or adult, speech community

Assimilation—the effect that one sound has on another when uttered close together, making the sounds alike; the result of coarticulation; adaptive articulatory changes by which one speech sound becomes similar, sometimes identical, to a neighboring speech sound

Coarticulation—the concept that the articulators are continually moving into position for other segments over a stretch of speech

Code mixing or code switching—when a speaker who speaks two languages, or dialects, shifts between the two, dependent on the situation or speaking context

Fossilized Forms—an incorrect production of a word that is not reflective of the child's current phonological abilities

Homonymy—the same pronunciation of two or more words that have different meanings

Idiosyncratic—unusual or atypical

Independent analysis—a description of a child's sound system as an independent, self-contained sound system; what a child can produce

IPA—International Phonetic Alphabet that contains the symbols used to represent the sounds in all natural languages of the world

Linguistics—all of the aspects pertaining to language, such as phonology, morphology, syntax, semantics, and pragmatics

Maximal oppositions—an intervention approach that contrasts the child's error with an independent sound that is maximally different from the target sound and is produced correctly by the child (Gierut, 1989)

Minimal Pair therapy—an intervention approach in which the target sound is contrasted with the child's error production for that sound; two words that differ by only one phoneme

Morphophonemic alternation—the occurrence of a different pronunciation of a phoneme when it occurs in a different morphemic context; for example, [dɑ] ~ [dɑgɪ] for "dog" ~ "doggie"

Multiple oppositions—an intervention approach that contrasts the child's error production for multiple target sounds that have been collapsed to the child's error sound (Williams, 2000)

Phonetic—production of sounds or phones; articulatory aspects of sound production

Phonemic—Sounds that are contrastive and signal a difference in meaning; the study of the sound system of language and the meaning of the sounds

Phonological disorder—a specific term used to describe error patterns of speech that reflect a linguistic, or phonemic, disorder in which the speech difficulties arise from differences in the development of phonological rules and in phonological organization relative to the ambient, or target, speech community

Phonological Process Analysis (PPA)—a method to describe and classify a child's error productions with regard to patterns or phonological processes, such as fronting, cluster reduction, et cetera

Phonotactics—the structural aspects of a sound system that specify the rules for combining phonemes in syllables and words of a specific language

Place-Voice-Manner Analysis (PVM)—a method to describe and classify a child's pattern of error productions on the basis of three broad categories of consonant production: place, voice, and manner

Relational analysis—a description and classification of a child's error productions relative to the adult target; also referred to as an error analysis

Speech delay—a term used to describe the slower speech development in children; generally about a year's delay

Speech differences—differences in speech that are characteristic of a particular linguistic or cultural group that are not considered a speech disorder

Speech disorder—a generic term used to describe both the phonetic and the phonemic aspects of speech disorders in children

Stimulability—the ability of a client to produce a sound when prompted or provided with auditory, visual, and tactile cues

Systemic Phonological Analysis of Child Speech (SPACS)—a method to describe the organization and rules that are present in a child's sound system by using independent and relational analyses that map the child:adult sound system in terms of phoneme collapses

Treatment of the empty set—an intervention approach that contrasts two unknown sounds that are maximally different (Gierut, 1991)

INTERNET RESOURCES

●●●

A listing of Internet sites has been compiled as an additional resource in working with children who have speech disorders. The sites are organized by topic area, and a brief description is provided.

GENERAL INFORMATION ON SPEECH AND LANGUAGE

www.SLPsite.com
This site is run by Dr. Caroline Bowen, an SLP from Australia. This Web site contains links to more than 184 Web pages. It contains useful information about communication disorders. It also has a "Site of the Month."

http://fonsg3.let.uva.nl/Reading_Room.html
This site is related to different reading material for speech and sound, and it also supplies a great source of references. It breaks down the material into phonetics, computer speech, signal processing, linguistics, other, and journals. This site also offers an online dictionary.

www.centerforspeech.com
This site is The Center for Speech, Language, and Learning homepage. The center is located in Houston, Texas. It has a "Kids Only" link that takes you to a colorful page filled with games and neat things for kids. The site also has a "Common Questions" link that takes you to a list of frequently asked questions about communication disorders.

www.angelfire.com/nj/speechlanguage/SLResources.html
This site is the homepage for Carol's Speech and Language Disorders Professional Resources. It provides information about specific speech and language disorders, articles that you might wish to share with clients or their parents, sample lesson plans, and examples of therapy materials. Some of the disorders featured include: apraxia, articulation, autism, cleft palate, dysphagia, phonological awareness, stuttering, and voice.

www.speechpaths.com

This site provides a community information resource for SLPs and audiologists. This site was designed to give the health care professionals a forum to exchange ideas and research information over the internet. Some of the features of this Web site include a "What's New?" section, an online "Bookstore," "Forums," and a "Kids Corner." The site also includes a "Continuing Education" section, which gives you the opportunity to complete continuing education credit hours online.

www.audiospeech.ubc.ca/eli/elimenu.htm

This resource site has information for Speech-Language Pathologists on Early Language Intervention. There is a "Fast Facts" section that gives useful facts about language development. There is a "Starters" section that gives core ideas for intervention activities. There is a "Research News" section that gives the latest findings on intervention. Finally, there is a "Books and Media" section that gives suggestions for your library. In each section, you can choose "Phonology" or "The Rest" of language.

www.advanceforspanda.com

This site is the homepage for ADVANCE magazine for Speech-Language Pathologists and Audiologists. You can search the magazine online for articles, online jobs, and continuing education events. This site also has several links to other useful Web sites.

www.mankato.msus.edu/dept/comdis/kuster2/splang.html

This site is an index of resources and information on the Internet that deal with speech-language deficits and disorders. Some topics included are: general information about communication disorders, child language disorders, adult language disorders, and voice disorders. This site is run by Judith Maginnis Kuster, who is an SLP and an associate professor at Minnesota State University, Mankato.

www.sphlangsys.com

This site is the homepage for Speech and Language Systems, Inc., located in Plymouth, Michigan. Speech and Language Systems, Inc. is a full-service pediatric rehabilitation agency with professionals in the fields of speech, physical, and occupational therapies and education. The site has links to pages that have more information about their specialized speech services such as "Fast-Forward," "Links-To-Language," and "Cued Speech." This site is run by Lorraine Zaksek, M.S., CCC, owner and director.

www.kidspeech.com

This site is the homepage for the Kaufman Children's Center for Speech and Language Disorders. The center is directed by Nancy R. Kaufman, M.A., CCC-SLP, who has more than 21 years of experience with the preschool population. The Web site has a section that highlights the services and specialties of the center. It also has a section with the testimonials of past clients and their parents and a section of helpful links to other Web sites.

www.healthtouch.com

This site is the Healthtouch Online homepage. If you take the "Health Information" link, then type "speech" to search, it comes up with four links: Children and Language, Language Development, Speech and Language Problems, and Communication Disorders. Each link takes you to areas of specific information about that topic. This site is a great general resource.

PHONOLOGY AND ARTICULATION

www.kidsource.com/ASHA/articulation.html
The KidSource site provides detailed consumer information on articulation disorders and links to related Web sites.

www.learningfundamentals.com/Phonology/Phonology.html
This Web site has descriptions of six games to play for phonological process therapy. Examples are: Minimal Pairs, Patterns, Word Practice, Match Ups, Word Blending, and What's Wrong. Each game has a link that takes you to a brief description of the activity. You can order the CD online from LocuTour Multimedia.

http://members.tripod.com/Caroline_Bowen/phonol-and-artic.htm
This site contains questions and answers about children's speech sound disorders. The questions are broken down into areas: Introduction: Phonology/Speech Development, Developmental Phonological Disorders, Functional Speech Disorders, Developmental Apraxia of Speech, The Dysarthrias, and Links. This site is featured in *The Therapist's Internet Handbook.*

www.quia.com/speech.html
This site contains activities created by SLPs for therapy. Most of the current activities are for articulation therapy. You can create your own activities and nominate activities for publication on the Web site. You can also review nominated activities.

www.speechtx.com
This site is the Speechtx store online homepage. This site has numerous activities and ideas for various ages that can be printed free. It has activities for articulation, language, and emergent literacy. The site also offers a CD for purchase that contains lots of activities and materials. You can view an online table of contents for the CD.

www.ling.udel.edu/idsardi/101/notes/phonology.html
This site is from William James Idsardi at the University of Delaware. This site has a great overview of the basics of phonology.

CHILD APRAXIA OF SPEECH / MOTOR SPEECH DISORDERS

www.apraxia-kids.org
This site is the official site for kids who have apraxia. This site has several useful sections. "Help!" is where you can find answers to your questions about apraxia. "Speech Topics" is where you can find most of the articles on the Web site, such as articles on therapy techniques written by top SLPs and how to find an experienced SLP. "Talk to Others" is where you can talk to other parents and SLPs via message boards, chat rooms, and e-mail. "News" is the section where you can read the latest apraxia news and see what is new on the Web site. This area is also where you can sign up for *The Apraxia-Kids Monthly* newsletter. "Recommended Resources" has links to other Web sites, information about books, and catalogs available. "FAQs" are articles written in a question and answer format. "About Us" tells you more about the people behind the Web site. "Articles By Author" are the same articles that are in

"Speech Topics," but here you can search for a specific author. Parents and caregivers write "Family Essays" about their experiences. "Search" enables you to search the Web site for a particular topic of interest. "Site Map" shows the layout of the Web site.

www.cs.Amherst.edu/~djv/DVD.html
This site gives parents basic information and gives professionals a bibliography of key articles and texts about developmental verbal dyspraxia.

www.ticeinfo.com/speech/index.html
This site contains large bibliographies of areas related to motor speech problems, including degenerative dysarthria, developmental apraxia, and so on. This site also carries links to related sites and a table of contents for the proceedings of the Speech Motor Control Conference.

INTERNATIONAL PHONETIC ASSOCIATION INFORMATION

http://www2.arts.gla.ac.uk/IPA/ipa.html
This site is the homepage for the International Phonetic Association (IPA). This site has links to the full IPA alphabet, diacritics, recordings of the sounds of the IPA, and the history of the IPA. The complete IPA handbook and also information on joining the IPA can be found here.

http://www2.arts.gla.ac.uk/IPA/cassettes.html
At this site, you can get an audiocassette and a CD of IPA sounds. Also available are downloadable audio files that accompany the language illustrations in the IPA handbook.

http://www.sil.org/computing/catalog/ipahelp.html
This site is another page with a free downloadable audio help chart. You can hear each IPA sound along with a language sample for each.

http://hctv.humnet.ucla.edu/departments/linguistics/VowelsandConsonants/
This Web site has audio information that goes along with Peter Ladefoged's books: *Vowels and Consonants* (Blackwells, 2001) and *A Course in Phonetics 4th Edition* (Harcourt College Publishers, 2000).

http://www2.arts.gla.ac.uk/IPA/ipafonts.html
This site has information about the different programs available for your computer containing IPA symbols. Some are free while others are available at a reasonable cost.

http://www.sil.org/computing/fonts/encore-ipa.html
At this site, you can download the SIL IPA fonts. These are available for Windows and Macintosh systems.

http://www.chass.utoronto.ca/~rogers/fonts.html
At this site, you can download the IPAPhon fonts. These are available for Windows and Macintosh systems.

PHONOLOGICAL AWARENESS

www.lblp.com/phonemicawareness.html
This site has a good description of phonemic awareness. It includes sections on the cause and symptoms that accompany problems with phonemic awareness. The solution they provide on this Web site is the Lindamood Phonemic Sequencing (LiPS) Program. This site also has programs available for the treatment of reading and spelling, comprehension, critical thinking, sight words, spelling, math, and visual motor problems. The site has information on instruction, testing, locations, workshops, school certification, multimedia resources, books and kits, and research. It also has a section for terms and definitions used on the Web site.

www.picturewordwall.com
This site is the homepage for Caboodle and Company Picture Word Wall and Balanced Booklets. These books are divided into four kits. Each kit contains reproducible, high-frequency lessons that teach the most useful words in the English language.

SPECIAL NEEDS POPULATIONS

www.unomaha.edu/~wwwsped/spd/apl/kas/tpc/a.html
This site is authored by Kathryn Shymanski, a Speech-Language Pathology major who works with toddlers who have Down syndrome. The site contains information about the language skills of individuals with cognitive impairments. It has sections of specific information on syntax, morphology, phonology, semantics, and pragmatics as they relate to individuals with cognitive impairments.

http://parentpals.com/4.0Teaching/teaching.html
This site provides a resource for parents of special education children. It offers special education games, products, and everyday tips to use at home.

REFERENCES

Aase, D., Hovic, C., Krause, K., Schelfhout, S., Smith, J. and Carpenter, L. (2000). *Contextual Test of Articulation.* Eau Claire: Thinking Publications.

Adams, C., Nighingale, C., Hesketh, A., and Hall, R. (2000). Targeting metaphonogical ability in intervention for children with developmental phonological disorders. *Child Language Teaching and Therapy*, 33(285–299).

Adams, M. (1990). *Beginning to read: Thinking and learning about print.* Cambridge, MA: MIT Press.

Aram, D. M., and Hall, N. E. (1989). Longitudinal follow-up of children with preschool communication disorders: Treatment implications. *School Psychology Review, 18,* 487–501.

ASHA. (2000). Communication facts. Science and Research Department, Rockville, MD: American Speech-Language-Hearing Association.

Bankson, N. and Bernthal, J. (1990). *Bankson-Bernthal Test of Phonology (BBTOP).* San Antonio: Riverside Publishing Co.

Bankson, N. W., and Bernthal, J. E. (1990). *Quickscreen of Phonology:* The Riverside Publishing Company.

Barlow, J. A., and Gierut, J. A. (1999). Optimality Theory in Phonological Acquisition. *Journal of Speech, Language, and Hearing Research, 42,* 1482–1498.

Bell, N. (1997). *Seeing Stars: Symbol imagery for phonemic awareness, sight words, and spelling.* San Luis Obiscop, CA: Gander.

Bello, J. (1995). *Prevalence of communication disorders among children in the United States.* Rockville: ASHA Science and Research Department.

Bernthal, J., and Bankson, N. (1998). *Articulation and phonological disorders (4th ed.).* Englewood Cliffs: Prentice-Hall.

Bird, J., Bishop, D. V. M., and Freeman, N. H. (1995). Phonological awareness and literacy development in children with expressive phonological impairments. *Journal of Child Psychology and Psychiatry, 31,* 1027–1050.

Blachman, B. (1984). Relationship of rapid naming ability and language analysis skill to kindergarten and first-grade reading achievement. *Journal of Educational Psychology, 76,* 610–622.

Blachman, B., Ball, E., Black, R., and Tangel, D. (2000). *Road to the code: A phonological awareness program for young children.* Baltimore, MD: Brookes.

Bleile, K. M. (1995). *Manual of articulation and phonological disorders: Infancy through adulthood.* Clifton Park, NY: Delmar Learning.

Bloom, M., and Fischer, J. (1982). *Evaluating practice: Guidelines for the accountable professional.* Englewood Cliffs, NJ: Prentice-Hall.

Bonderman, I. R. (1986). A preschool program for severe phonological disorders: A handbook for speech and language pathologists., Fountain Valley School District.

Burns, S. M., Griffin, P., and Snow, C. E. (1999). *Starting out right: A guide to promoting children's reading success.* National Academy Press: Washington, D.C.

Camarata, S. M. (1993). The application of naturalistic conversation training to speech production in children with speech disabilities. *Journal of Applied Behavior Analysis, 26,* 173–182.

Camarata, S. M. (1995). A rationale for naturalistic speech intelligibility intervention. *Language intervention: Preschool through the elementary years, 63*–84.

Camarata, S. M., and Gandour, J. (1984). On describing idiosyncratic phonological systems. *Journal of Speech and Hearing Disorders, 49,* 262–265.

Carrow, E. (1974). *Austin Spanish Articulation Test (ASAT):* Teaching Resources.

Carter, E. T., and Buck, M. W. (1958). Prognostic testing for functional articulation disorders among children in the first grade. *Journal of Speech and Hearing Disorders, 23,* 124–133.

Catts, H. W. (1991). Facilitating phonological awareness: Role of speech-language pathologists. *Language, Speech, and Hearing Services in Schools, 26,* 196–203.

Catts, H. W. (1993). The relationship between speech-language impairments and reading disabilities. *Journal of Speech and Hearing Disorders, 36,* 948–958.

Catts, H. W. (1997). The early identification of language-based reading disabilities. *Language, Speech, and Hearing Services in Schools, 28,* 86–87.

Catts, H. W., and Vartiainen. (1996). *Sounds Abound Game.* East Moline: LinguiSystems.

Chomsky, N., and Halle, M. (1968). *The sound pattern of English.* New York: Harper and Row.

Clark-Klein, S., and Hodson, B. W. (1995). A phonologically based analysis of misspellings by third graders with disordered-phonology histories. *Journal of Speech and Hearing Disorders, 38,* 839–849.

Cole, P. A., and Taylor, O. L. (1990). Performance of working class African-American children on three tests of articulation. *Language, Speech, and Hearing Services in Schools, 21,* 171–176.

Compton, A. J., and Hutton, S. (1978). *Compton-Hutton phonological assessment.* San Francisco: Carousel House.

Connolly, J. H. (1986). Intelligibility: A linguistic view. *British Journal of Disorders of Communication, 21,* 371–376.

Costello, J. M. (1979). Clinicians and researchers: A necessary dichotomy? *Journal of the National Student Speech-Hearing Association, 7,* 6–26.

Culatta, B. and Horn, D. (1982). A program for achieving generalization of grammatical rules to spontaneous discourse. *Journal of Speech and Hearing Disorders, 47,* 174–180.

Davis, B. L., Jakielski, K. T., and Marquardt, T. P. (1998). Developmental apraxia of speech: Determiners of differential diagnosis. *Clinical Linguistics and Phonetics, 12,* 25–45.

Di Simoni, F. (1978). *The Token Test for Children:* Hingham Teaching Resources Corporation.

Dinnsen, D. A. and Elbert, M. (1984). On the relationship between phonology and learning. *Phonological theory and the misarticulating child.* Rockville, MD: American Speech-Language-Hearing Association.

Dinnsen, D. A., Gierut, J. A., and Chin, S. (1987). Underlying representations and the differentiation of functional misarticulators. Paper presented at the annual meeting of the American Speech-Language-Hearing Association, New Orleans, LA.

Dinnsen, D. A., Gierut, J. A., and Chin, S. (1987). *Underlying representations and the differentiation of functional misarticulations.* Paper presented at the annual meeting of the American Speech-Language Hearing Association. New Orleans, LA.

Drumwright, A. F., and Frankenburg, W. K. (1971). *Denver Articulation Screening Exam:* Denver Developmental Materials, INC.

Dunn, C. (1982). Phonological process analysis: Contributions to assessing phonological disorders. *Communicative Disorders, 7,* 147–164.

Dunn, L. M., and Dunn, L. M. (1981). *Peabody picture vocabulary test-revised.* Circle Pines: American Guidance System.

Education, W. C. B. o. (1995). *The Phonological Awareness Companion: Making the Speech-Print Connection.* East Moline: LinguiSystems.

Edwards, M. L. (1994). In support of phonological processes: Clinical forum: Phonological assessment and treatment. *Language, Speech, and Hearing Services in Schools, 23,* 233–240.

Edwards, M. L. (1994). Phonological process analysis. In *Children's phonological disorders,* Rockville, MD: American Speech-Language-Hearing Association, 43–65.

Elbert, M. (1992). Consideration of error types: A response to Fey. Clinical Forum: Phonological assessment and treatment. *Language, Speech, and Hearing Services in Schools, 23,* 241–246.

Elbert, M., Dinnsen, D. A., and Powell, T. W. (1984). On the prediction of phonological generalization learning pattern. *Journal of Speech and Hearing Disorders, 49,* 309–317.

Elbert, M, and Gierut, J. A. (1986). *Handbook of clinical phonology: Approaches to assessment and treatment.* San Diego, CA: College-Hill Press.

Elbert, M, and McReynolds, L. V. (1978). An experimental analysis of misarticulation children's generalization. *Journal of Speech and Hearing Research, 21,* 136–150.

Elbert, M., Rockman, B. K., and Saltzman, D. (1980). *Contrasts: The use of minimal pairs in articulation and treatment.* Austin: Exceptional Resources.

Fazio, B. B., and Williams, A. L. (1989). *Parents as members of a language intervention team. Paper presented at the ASHA convention.* St. Louis, MO.

Felsenfeld, S., Broen, P. A., and McGue, M. (1994). A 28-year follow-up of adults with a history of moderate phonological disorder: Educational and occupational results. *Journal of Speech and Hearing Disorders, 37,* 1341–1353.

Fenson, L., Dale, P. S., Reznick, S., Thal, D., Bates, E., Hartung, J., Pethick, J., and Reilly, J. (1993). *MacArthur Communicative Development Inventories.* Clifton Park, NY: Delmar Learning.

Ferrier, E., and Davis, M. (1973). A lexical approach to the remediation of final sound omissions. *Journal of Speech and Hearing Disorders, 38,* 126–130.

Fey, M. E. (1986). *Language intervention with young children.* Boston: Allyn & Bacon.

Fey, M. E. (1992). Articulation and phonology: Inextricable constructs in speech pathology. Clinical Forum: Phonological assessment and treatment. *Language, Speech, and Hearing Services in Schools, 23,* 225–232.

Fey, M. E., Catts, H. W., and Larrivae, L. S. (1995). Preparing preschoolers for the academic and social challenges of school., *Language Intervention: Preschool through the elementary years.* (pp. 3–37). Baltimore, MD: Paul H. Brookes Publishing Company.

Fey, M. E., Cleave, P. L., Ravida, A. I., Long, S. H., Gegmal, A. E., and Easton, D. L. (1994). Effects of grammar facilitation on the phonological performance of children with speech and language impairments. *Journal of Speech and Hearing Research, 37,* 594–607.

Fisher, H. and Logemann, J. (1971). *Fisher-Logemann Test of Articulation Competence.* Boston: Houghton-Mifflin.

Fluharty, N. B. (1978). *Fluharty Preschool Speech and Language Screening Test.* Danville: Pro-Ed.

Forrest, K. (2002). Are oral-motor exercises useful in the treatment of phonological/articulatory disorders? *Seminars in Speech and Language, 23(1),* 15–25.

Forrest, K., and Morrisette, M. L. (1999). Feature analysis of segmental errors in children with phonological disorders. *Journal of Speech nd Hearing Research, 42,* 187–194.

Fudala, J., and Reynolds, W. (1986). *Arizona Articulation Proficiency Scale-2nd Edition (AAPA-2).* Los Angeles: Western Psychological Services.

Gardner, M. F. (1990). *Expressive One-Word Picture Vocabulary Test.* Novato: Academic Therapy Publications.

German, D. J. (2000). *Test of Word Finding-2.* Austin, TX: PROED.

Gierut, J. A. (1985). On the relationship between phonological knowledge and generalization learning in misarticulating children., Doctoral dissertation, Indiana University: Bloomington.

Gierut, J. A. (1986). On the assessment of productive phonological knowledge. *Journal of the National Student Speech-Hearing Association, 14,* 83–100.

Gierut, J. A. (1989). Maximal opposition approach to phonological treatment. *Journal of Speech and Hearing Disorders, 54,* 9–19.

Gierut, J. A. (1990). Differential learning of phonological oppositions. *Journal of Speech and Hearing Research, 33,* 540–549.

Gierut, J. A. (1991). Homonymy in Phonological Change. *Clinical Linguistics and Phonetics, 5,* 119–137.

Gierut, J. A. (1992). The conditions and course of clinically induced phonological change. *Journal of Speech and Hearing Research, 35,* 1049–1063.

Gierut, J. A. (1998). Treatment efficacy: Functional phonological disorders in children. *Journal of speech, Language, and Hearing Research, 41,* s85–s100.

Gierut, J. A., Elbert, M., and Dinnsen, D. A. (1987). A functional analysis of phonological knowledge and generalization learning in misarticulating children. *Journal of Speech and Hearing Research, 30,* 462–479.

Gierut, J. A., Morrisett, M. L., Hughes, M. T., and Rowland, S. (1996). Phonological treatment efficacy and developmental norms. *Language, Speech, and Hearing Services in the Schools, 27,* 215–230.

Gillon, G. T. (2000). The efficacy of phonological awareness intervention for children with spoken language impairment. *Language, Speech, and Hearing Services in Schools, 31,* 126–141.

Goldman, and Fristoe. (2000). *Goldman-Fristoe Test of Articulation-2.* Circle Pines: American Guidance Service.

Goldman, R., and Fristoe, M. (1986). *Goldman-Fristoe test of articulation.* Circle Pines: American Guidance Service.

Goldsmith, J. (1976). An overview of autosegmental phonology. *Linguistic Analysis, 2,* 23–68.

Goldsmith, J. (1976). *Autosegmental phonology.,* Ph.D. dissertation, Massachusetts Institute of Technology (published by Garland Press, 1979).

Goldsmith, J. (1990). Autosegmental and Metrical phonology. *Lingua, 80,* 375.

Goldsmith, J. A. (1990). *Autosegmental and metrical phonology.* Osford: Basil Blackwell.

Goldstein, B. (2000). *Cultural and linguistic diversity: Resource guide for speech-language pathologists.* Clifton Park, NY: Delmar Learning.

Gordon-Brannan, M., Hodson, B. W., and Wynne, M. (1992). Remediating unintelligible utterances of a child with a mild hearing loss. *American Journal of Speech-Language Pathology, 1,* 28–38.

Grunwell, P. (1986). *Phonological Assessment of Child Speech.* San Diego: College-Hill Press.

Grunwell, P. (1987). *Clinical Phonology (2nd ed.).* London: Croom Helm.

Grunwell, P. (1997). Developmental phonological disability: Order in disorder. *Perspectives in applied phonology,* Gaithersburg, MD: Aspen Publications.

Hall, P. K. (2000). A letter to the parent(s) of a child with developmental apraxia of speech, Part IV: Treatment of DAS. *Language, Speech, and Hearing Services in Schools, 31,* 179–181.

Hall, P. K., Jordon, L. S., and Robin, D. A. (1993). *Developmental apraxia of speech: Theory and clinical practice.* Austin, TX: PRO-ED.

Hendrick, D. L., Prather, E. M., and Tobin, A. R. (1984). *Sequence Inventory of Communication Development Revised Edition.* Austin, TX: PROED.

Hodson, B. W. (1985). *Computerized Assessment of Phonological Processes (CAPP):* Interstate Printers and Publishers.

Hodson, B. W. (1986). *Assessment of phonological processes-revised.* Austin: Pro-Ed.

Hodson, B. W. (1986). *Assessment of Phonological Processes-Revised (APP-R).* Danville: Pro-Ed.

Hodson, B. W. (1986). *Assessment of Phonological Process-Spanish (APP-S):* Los Amigos Association.

Hodson, B. W. (1992). Applied phonology: constructs, contributions, and issues. Clinical Forum: Phonological assessment and treatment. *Language, Speech, and Hearing Services in Schools, 23,* 247–253.

Hodson, B. W. (1998). Research and Practice: Applied Phonology. *Topics in Language Disorders, 18*(2), 58–70.

Hodson, B. W., Chin, L., Redmond, B., and Simpson, R. (1983). Phonological evaluation and remediation of speech deviations of a child with a repaired cleft palate: A case study. *Journal of Speech and Hearing Disorders, 48,* 93–98.

Hodson, B. W. and Paden, E. (1983). *Targeting intelligible speech.* San Diego: College-Hill.

Hodson, B. W., and Paden, E. (1991). *Targeting intelligible speech: A phonological approach to remediation* (2nd ed.). Austin, TX: Pro-Ed.

Hoffman, P. R., Norris, J. A., and Monjure, J. (1990). Comparison of process targeting and whole language treatment for phonologically delayed preschool children. *Language, Speech, and Hearing Services in Schools, 21,* 102–109.

Hresko, W. P., Herron, S. R., and Peak, P. K. (1996). *Test of Early Written Language.* Austin: Pro-Ed.

Iglesias, A., and Goldstein, B. (1998). Dialectal variations. In J. Bernthal and N. B. (Eds.) (Eds.), *Articulation and phonological disorders (4th ed.) (pp. 148–171).* Needham Heights, MA: Allyn & Bacon.

Ingram, D. (1997). The categorization of phonological impairment. *Perspectives in applied phonology.,* Gaithersburg, MD: Aspen Publications. 19–42.

Irwin, J. V., and Weston, A. J. (1971). *Paired Stimuli Kit.* Milwaukee, WI: Fox Point.

Johnston, J. R. (1984). Fit, focus, and functionality: An essay on early language intervention. *Child Language Teaching and Therapy, 1,* 125–134.

Kamhi, A. G., Allen, M. M., and Catts, H. W. (2001). The role of the speech-language pathologist in improving decoding skills. *Seminars in Speech and Language, 22,* 175–183.

Kent, R. D. (2000). A longitudinal case study of ALS: Effects of listener familiarity and proficiency on intelligibility judgments. *American Journal of Speech-Language Pathology, 3,* 230–240.

Kent, R. D., Miolo, G., and Bloedel, S. (1994). The intelligibility of children's speech: A review of evaluation procedures. *American Journal of Speech-Language Pathology, 3,* 81–95.

Khan, L. and Lewis, N. (1986). *Khan-Lewis Phonological Analysis:* AGS.

Kinzler, M. C. (1992). *Joliet 3-Minute Preschool Speech and Language Screen.:* Communication Skill Builders.

Kinzler, M. C., and Johnson, C. C. (1992). *Joliet 3-Minute Speech and Language Screen (Revised):* The Psychology Corporation.

Laney, M. (1982). Research and evaluation in the public schools. *Language, Speech, and Hearing Services in Schools, 13,* 53–60.

Leonard, L. B., and Brown, B. W. (1984). Nature and boundaries of phonologic categories: A case study of an unusual phonologic pattern in a language-impaired child. *Journal of Speech and Hearing Disorders, 49,* 419–428.

Lindamood, C. H., and Lindamood, P. C. (1971). *Lindamood Auditory Conceptualization Test.* Boston: Teaching Resources Corporation.

Long, S. H., and Fey, M. E. (1994). *Computerized Profiling.* Psychological Corporation.

Lowe, R. J. (1995). *Assessment Link Between Phonology and Articulation: Phonology Test Revised (ALPA):* ALPHA Speech & Language Resources.

Masterson, J., and Pagan, F. (1992). *Macintosh Interactive System for Phonological Analysis (ISPA):* Psychological Corporation.

Mattes, L. (1994). *Spanish Articulation Measures-Revised.* Academic Communication Associates.

Maxwell, E. M., and Rockman, B. K. (1984). Analysis of misarticulated speech. In D. A. D. M. Elbert, and G. Weismer (Eds.) (Ed.), *Phonological theory and the misarticulating child.* (ASHA Monographs No. 22, Ch. 7, pp. 69–91).

McCarthy, L. (1988). Feature geometry and dependency: A review. *Journal of Phonetics, 43,* 84–108.

McCune-Nicolich, L., and Carroll, S. (1981). Development of symbolic play: Implications for the language specialist. *Topics in Language Disorders, 1,* 1–15.

McDonald, E. (1964). *Deep test of articulation.* Pittsburgh, PA: Stanwix Heuse.

McReynolds, L. V., and Bennett, S. (1972). Distinctive feature generalization in articulations training. *Journal of Speech and Hearing Disorders, 37,* 462–470.

McReynolds, L. V., and Jetzke, E. (1986). Articulation generalization of voiced-voiceless sounds in hearing-impaired children. *Journal of Speech and Hearing Disorders, 51,* 348–355.

McReynolds, L. V., and Kearns, K. P. (1983). Single-subject experimental designs in communicative disorders. Baltimore: University Park.

Mecham, M. J., Jex, J. L., and Jones, J. D. (1970). *Screening Speech Articulation Test:* Communication Research Associates, INC.

Miccio, A. W., Elbert, M., and Forrest, K. (1999). The relationship between stimulability and phonological acquisition in children with normally developing and disordered phonologies. *American Journal of Speech-Language Pathology, 8,* 347–363.

Monaha, B. D. (1991). *Remediation of common phonological processes* (2nd ed.). Austin, TX: Pro-Ed, Inc.

Newcomer, P. L., and Hammill, D. D. (1997). *Test of language development primary-3.* Austin: Pro-ed.

Odell, K. H., and Shriberg, L. D. (2001). Prosody-voice characteristics of children and adults with apraxia of speech. *Clinical Linguistics and Phonetics, 15*(4), 275–308.

Oller, D. K., and Delgado, R. (1990). *Logical International Phonetic Programs (LIPP):* Intelligent Hearing Systems.

Olswang, L. B. (1990). Treatment efficacy research: A path to quality assurance. *ASHA, 32,* 45–47.

Palin, M. W. (1992). *Contrast pairs for phonological training.* Chicago, IL: The Riverside Publishing Company.

Panel, N.R. (2000). Children to read: An evidence based assessment of the scientific research literature on reading and its implications for reading instruction (NIH Pub. No. 00-4769). Washington, D.C.: National Institute of Child Health and Human Development.

Paradis, C. (1988). On constraints and repair strategies. *The Linguistic Review, 6,* 71–97.

Paul, R., and Jennings, P. (1992). Phonological Behaviors in Toddlers with Slow Expressive Language Development. *Journal of Speech and Hearing Disorders, 39,* 153–165.

Pendergrast, K., Dickey, S., Selma, J., and Soder, A. (1984). *Photo Articulation Test-2nd Edition (PAT-2).* Danville: Pro-Ed.

Perkins, W. H. (1985). From clinical dispenser to clinical scientist. *Seminars in Speech and Language, 6,* 13–21.

Powell, T. W. (2001). Phonetic transcription of disordered speech. *Topics in Language Disorders, 21*(4), 52–72.

Powell, T. W., Elbert, M., and Dinnsen, D. A. (1991). Stimulability as a factor in the phonological generalization of misarticulating preschool children. *Journal of Speech and Hearing Research, 34,* 1318–1328.

Prather, E., Hedrick, D., and Kern, C. (1975). Articulation development in children aged two to four years. *Journal of Speech and Hearing Disorders, 40,* 179–191.

Proctor, A. (1994). Phonology and cultural diversity. *Phonology: Assessment and intervention applications in speech pathology*, Baltimore: Williams & Wilkins. 207–245.

Reid, D. K., Hresko, W. P., and Hammill, D. D. (1989). *Test of Early Reading Ability.* Austin: Pro-Ed.

Rescorla, L., and Ratner, N. B. (1996). Phonetic Profiles of toddlers with specific expressive language development (SLI-E). *Journal of Speech and Hearing Research, 39,* 153–165.

Rice, M. L., Hadley, P. A., and Alexander, A. L. (1993). Social biases toward children with speech and language impairment: A correclative causal model of language limitations. *Applied Psycholinguistics, 14,* 445–471.

Robertson, C., and Salter, W. (1995). *The Phonological Awareness Profile.* East Moline: LinguiSystems, INC.

Robertson, C., and Salter, W. (1995). *Phonological Awareness Kit.* East Moline: LinguaSystems.

Robertson, C., and Salter, W. (1997). *The Phonological Awareness Test.* East Moline: LinguiSystems.

Rockman, B. K., and Elbert, M. (1984). Untrained acquisition of /s/ in a phonologically disordered child. *Journal of Speech and Hearing Disorders, 49,* 246–253.

Rosenbek, J. C., and Wertz, R. T. (1992). A review of fifty cases of developmental apraxia of speech. *Language, Speech, and Hearing Services in Schools, 3,* 23–33.

Roth, F. P., and Baden, B. (2001). Investing in emergent literacy intervention: A key role for speech-language pathologists. *Seminars in Speech and Language, 22*(3), 163–173.

Rvachew, S., and Nowak, M. (2001). The effect of phonological learning. *Journal of Speech, Language, and Hearing Research, 44,* 610–623.

Saben, C. B., and Ingham, J. C. (1991). The effects of minimal pairs treatment on the speech-sound production of two children with phonological disorders. *Journal of Speech and Hearing Research, 34,* 1023–1040.

Safer, N. D., and Hamilton, J. L. (1993). Legislative context for early intervention services. *Family-centered early intervention with infants and toddlers: Innovative cross-disciplinary approaches.,* Baltimore, Brookes Publishing Co.

Sagey, E. (1986). *The representation of features and relations in non-linear phonology.,* Unpublished Ph.D. dissertation, Massachusetts Institute of Technology, Cambridge, MA.

Sander, E. (1972). When are speech sounds learned? *Journal of Speech and Hearing Disorders, 37,* 55–63.

Schwartz, R., and Leonard, L. B. (1982). Do children pick and choose? An examination of phonological selection and avoidance in early lexical acquisition. *Journal of Child Language, 9,* 319–336.

Secord, W. (1981). *Test of Minimal Articulation Competence (T-MAC).* Columbus: Psychological Corporation.

Shriberg, L. D., and Kent, R. D. (1995). *Clinical phonetics.* Boston: Allyn & Bacon.

Shriberg, L. D. (1982). Toward classification of developmental phonological disorders. *Speech and Language: Advances in basic research and practice,* Austin, TX: Pro-Ed. 2–18.

Shriberg, L. D. (1986). *Programs to Examine Phonetic and Phonologic Evaluation Records (PEP-PER):* Lawrence Erlbaum.

Shriberg, L. D. (1993). Four new speech and prosody-voice measures for genetics research and other studies in developmental phonological disorders. *Journal of Speech and Hearing Research, 36,* 105–140.

Shriberg, L. D. (1994). Five subtypes of developmental phonological disorders. *Clinics in Communication Disorders, 41,* 38–45.

Shriberg, L. D. (1997). Developmental phonological disorders I: A clinical profile. *Journal of Speech and Hearing Disorders, 37,* 1100–1126.

Shriberg, L. D., and Kwiatkowski, J. (1980). *Natural Process Analysis (NPA):* John Wiley.

Shriberg, L. D., and Kwiatkowski, J. (1982). Phonological Disorders III: A procedure for assessing severity of involvement. *Journal of Speech and Hearing Disorders, 47,* 256–270.

Smit, A. B., and Hand, L. (1996). *Smit-Hand Articulation and Phonology Evaluation (SHAPE).* Los Angeles: Western Psychological Services.

Smit, A. B., Hand, L., Freilinger, J. J., Bernthal, J. E., and Bird, A. (1990). The Iowa articulation norms project and its Nebraska replication. *Journal of Speech and Hearing Research, 55,* 779–798.

Sparrow, S. S., Balla, D. A., and Cicchetti, D. V. (1984). *Vineland Adaptive Behavior Scales.* Circle Pines: American Guidance Service.

St. Louis, K. O., and Ruscello, D. M. (1997). *Oral Speech Mechanism Screening Examination, Third Edition.* Danville: Pro-Ed.

Stackhouse, J. (1997). Phonological awareness: Connecting speech and literacy problems. In B. W. Hodson and M. L. E. (Eds.) (Eds.), *Perspectives in applied phonology* (pp. 157–196). Gaithersburg, MD: Aspen Publishers, Inc.

Stanovich, K. E. (1986). Matthew effect in reading: Some consequences of individual differences in the acquisition of literacy. *Reading Research Quarterly, 21,* 360–407.

Stoel-Gammon, C. (1985). Phonetic inventories, 15–24 months: A longitudinal study. *Journal of Speech and Hearing Research, 28,* 506–512.

Stoel-Gammon C. (1987). Phonological skills in two-year-olds. *Language, Speech, and Hearing Services in Schools, 18,* 323–329.

Stoel-Gammon C. (1989). Prespeech and early speech development of two late talkers. *First Language, 9,* 207–224.

Stoel-Gammon C. (1991). Normal and disordered phonology in two-year-olds. *Topics in Language Disorders, 11,* 21–32.

Templin, M., and Darley, F. L. (1969). *Templin-Darley Test of Articulation.* Iowa City: Speech Bin.

Torgeson, J. K., and Bryant, B. R. (1994). *Test of Phonological Awareness.* Austin: Pro-Ed.

Turton, C. J. (1973). Diagnostic implications of articulation testing. *Articulation and learning,* Springfield, IL: Charles C. Thomas. 195–232.

Tyler, A. A., Edwards, M. L., and Saxman, J. H. (1990). Acoustic validation of phonological knowledge and its relationship to treatment. *Journal of Speech and Hearing Disorders, 55,* 251–261.

Tyler, A. A., and Sandoval, K. T. (1994). Preschoolers with phonological and language disorders: Treating different linguistic domains. *Language, Speech, and Hearing Services in Schools, 25,* 215–234.

Van Kleeck, A., Gillam, R. B., and McFadden, T. U. (1998). A study of classroom-based phonological awareness training for preschoolers with speech and/or language disorders. *American Journal of Speech-Language Pathology, 7,* 65–76.

Van Riper, C. (1939). *Speech correction: Principles and methods.* Englewood Cliffs, NJ: Prentice Hall.

Wagner, R. K., Torgeson, J. K., and Rashotte. (1999). *Comprehensive Test of Phonological Processing.* Austin: Pro-Ed.

Wasowicz, J. (1998). *Earobics Auditory Development and Phonics Program.* Evanston: Cognitive Concepts.

Watts, S. A., and Payneter, E. T. (1973). Watts Articulation Test for Screening: Evaluation of a screening test. *Perceptual and Motor Skills, 36,* 721–722.

Weber, J. L. (1970). Patterning of deviant articulation behavior. *Journal of Speech and Hearing Disorders, 35,* 135–141.

Weiner, F. (1979). *Phonological Process Analysis.* Danville: Pro-Ed.

Weiner, F. (1981). Treatment of phonological disability using the methods of meaningful minimal contrast: Two case studies. *Journal of Speech and Hearing Disorders, 46,* 97–103.

Weiner, F. (1982). *Phonological process analysis.* Austin: Pro-Ed.

Weiner, F., and Bankson, N. (1978). Teaching Features. *Language, Speech, and Hearing Services in Schools, 9,* 29–34.

Weiss, C. (1980). *Weiss Comprehensive Articulation Test:* Pro-Ed.

Weston, A. D., and Shriberg, L.D. (1992). Contextual and linguistic correlates of intelligibility in children with developmental phonological disorders. *Journal of Speech and Hearing Research, 35,* 1316–1332.

Wiig, E. H., Secord, W., and Semel, E. (1995). *Clinical Evaluation of Language Fundamentals—3.* San Antonio: Psychological Corporation.

Williams, A. L. (1991). Generalization patterns associated with training least phonological knowledge. *Journal of Speech and Hearing Research,* 34, 722–733.

Williams, A. L. (1992). Multiple oppositions: An alternative contrastive therapy approach., Paper presented at the meeting of the American Speech-Language-Hearing Association, San Antonio, TX.

Williams, A. L. (1993a). Phonological reorganization: A qualitative measure of phonological improvement. *American Journal of Speech-Language Pathology, 2,* 44–51.

Williams, A. L. (1993b). The use of single-subject designs in clinical practice. *Clinics in Communication Disorders, 3(3),* 47-58.

Williams, A. L. (1995). Modified teaching clinic: Peer group supervision in clinical training and professional development. *American Journal of Speech-Language Pathology, 4,* 29–38.

Williams, A. L. (2000a). Multiple oppositions: Theoretical foundations for an alternative contrastive intervention approach. *American Journal of Speech-Language Pathology, 9,* 282–288.

Williams, A. L. (2000b). Multiple oppositions: Case studies of variables in phonological intervention. *American Journal of Speech-Language Pathology, 9,* 289–299.

Williams, A. L. (2001). Phonological assessment of child speech. *Tests and Measurements in Speech-Language Pathology.,* D. M. Ruscello (Ed.). Woburn MA: Butterworth-Heinemann.

Williams, A. L., and Dinnsen, D. A. (1987). A problem of allophonic variation in a speech disordered child. *Innovations in Linguistic Education, 5(1),* 85–90.

Williams, A. L. and Elbert, M. (2002). A prospective longitudinal study of phonological development in late talkers. Manuscript in preparation.

Williams, A. L., and Kalbfleisch, J. (2001). *Phonological intervention using a multiple opposition approach.* Paper presented at the 25th World Congress of the International Association of Logopedics and Phoniatrics, Montreal, Canada.

Yopp, H. K. (1992). Developing phonemic awareness young children. *Reading Teacher, 45,* 696–703.

Yorkston, K. M., Beukelman, D. R., Stand, E. A., and Bell, K. R. (1999). *Management of motor speech disorders in children and adults (2nd ed.).* Austin, TX: Pro-Ed.

Yoss, K. A., and Darley, F. L. (1974). Developmental apraxia of speech in children with defective articulation. *Journal of Speech and Hearing Research, 17,* 399–416.

Zimmerman, I. L., Steiner, V. G., and Pond, R. e. (1992). *Preschool Language Scale—3:* The Psychological Corporation.

INDEX

Note: Boldface numbers indicate illustrations.